T0276498

Diagnosis, Prevention and Management of T-Cell Leukemia

Diagnosis, Prevention and Management of T-Cell Leukemia

Edited by **George Singer**

New Jersey

Published by Foster Academics,
61 Van Reypen Street,
Jersey City, NJ 07306, USA
www.fosteracademics.com

Diagnosis, Prevention and Management of T-Cell Leukemia
Edited by George Singer

International Standard Book Number: 978-1-63242-116-6 (Hardback)

Printed in the United States of America.

Contents

Preface

An elucidative account regarding the diagnosis, prevention and management of T-cell leukemia has been presented in this book. T-cell leukemia is a comparatively rare malignancy of thymocytes. Nearly 20 variants and entities of this disease are known to exist. Each one of them has distinct characteristics, like diagnosis, pathogenesis, prognosis, epidemiology and therapeutic approaches. Although it is a relatively rare malignancy, various types of T-cell leukemia still result in a poor prognosis due to their quick progression. Hence, growth in new preventive and therapeutic strategies is required for improving prognosis. The aim of this book is to present the readers with a descriptive study of the disease encompassing the basics of epidemiology, immunological features, pathogenesis and morphology. The book also emphasizes on the current achievements in fundamental and clinical researches including new therapies and molecular mechanisms of T-cell leukemia.

This book is a result of research of several months to collate the most relevant data in the field.

When I was approached with the idea of this book and the proposal to edit it, I was overwhelmed. It gave me an opportunity to reach out to all those who share a common interest with me in this field. I had 3 main parameters for editing this text:

1. Accuracy – The data and information provided in this book should be up-to-date and valuable to the readers.
2. Structure – The data must be presented in a structured format for easy understanding and better grasping of the readers.
3. Universal Approach – This book not only targets students but also experts and innovators in the field, thus my aim was to present topics which are of use to all.

Thus, it took me a couple of months to finish the editing of this book.

I would like to make a special mention of my publisher who considered me worthy of this opportunity and also supported me throughout the editing process. I would also like to thank the editing team at the back-end who extended their help whenever required.

Editor

Molecular Morphogenesis of T-Cell Acute Leukemia

Michael Litt, Bhavita Patel, Ying Li, Yi Qiu and
Suming Huang

Additional information is available at the end of the chapter

1. Introduction

Many molecular alterations are involved in the morphogenesis of T-cell acute leukemia (T-ALL), classified as lymphoblastic leukemia/lymphoma by the World Health Organization. T-ALL is a malignant disease of the thymocytes which accounts for approximately 15% of pediatric acute lymphoblastic leukemia (ALL) and 20-25% of adult ALL. Frequently, it presents with a high tumor load accompanied by rapid disease progression. About 30% of T-ALL cases relapse within the first two years following diagnosis with long term remission in 70-80% of children and 40% of adults [1]-[4]. This poor prognosis is a consequent of our insufficient knowledge of the molecular mechanisms underlying abnormal T-cell pathogenesis. Understanding the abnormal molecular changes associated with T-ALL biology will provide us with the tools for better diagnosis and treatment of lymphoblastic leukemia. Recent improvements in genome-wide profiling methods have identified several genetic aberrations which are associated with T-ALL pathogenesis. For simplification these molecular changes can be separated into 4 different groups: chromosome aberrations, gene mutations, gene expression profiles, and epigenetic alterations. This chapter will discuss these molecular changes in depth.

2. T-cell development

The progenitors for T lymphocytes arise in the bone marrow as long-term repopulating hematopoietic stem cells (LT-HSCs) (Figure 1). These cells then differentiate, generating short-term repopulating hematopoietic stem cells (ST-HSCs) and lymphoid-primed multipotent progenitor (LMPP)[5]-[7]. LMPPs, which migrate via the blood and a chemotaxis process to the thymus [8], phenotypically resemble early T-cell progenitors (ETP)[9],[10]. ETP cells, also called double negative 1 (DN1), are capable of differentiating into either T-cells or myeloid cells and phenotypically belong to a CD3⁻CD4⁻/lowCD8⁻CD25⁻CD44⁻KIT⁺ (Figures 1 and 2). If ETP cells commit to the T-cell lineage they progress to double negative 2 (DN2), followed by double negative 3 (DN3) and finally double negative 4 (DN4) T-cell development stages. This process starts with the downregulation of c-KIT receptor resulting in the cell surface phenotype CD4⁻CD8⁻CD25⁺CD44⁻ for DN2 cells, next CD44 is lost for a cell surface phenotype of CD4⁻CD8⁻CD25⁺CD44⁻ for DN3 cells, and finally CD25 is lost for a cell surface phenotype of CD4⁻CD8⁻CD25⁻CD44⁻ for DN4 cells (Figures 1 and 2) [9],[11]-[13]. This differentiation from ETP to DN4 cells occurs within the thymus in intimate contact with the epithelial stromal cells, which express Notch ligands, essential growth factors (interleukin-7), and morphogens (sonic hedgehog proteins) important for T-cell development. Before differentiation into double positive cells (DP) which have the cell surface phenotype CD4⁺CD8⁺, DN4 cells lose their dependence on Notch ligand, interleukin-7 and sonic hedgehog (Shh) [14],[15]. Once they are DP cells, they undergo positive and negative selection. Following selection, αβ T-cell receptor (TCR)⁺ T cells migrate from the thymus to secondary lymphoid organs to manifest their immune function. These mature cells are single positive (SP) with the cell surface phenotype of either CD4⁺ or CD8⁺ [9],[11].

T-cell Development

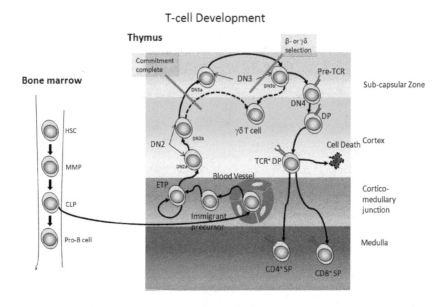

Figure 1. Stages in T-cell development. The different regions of the adult thymic lobule are indicated to the rights. The progression of hematopoietic stem cells (HSC), multipotent progenitors (MPP), and the common lymphoid progenitors (CLPs) are shown to the left in the bone marrow. Lymphoid progenitors migrated through the blood to the thymus. The migration and differentiation from immigrant precursor to early T-cell precursors (ETP), to double negative (DN), to double positive (DP), and to single positive (SP) stages is illustrated within the distinct microenvironments of the thymus. Complete commitment to the T-cell lineage is indicated with a line between the DN2b and DN3a stages. β or γδ selection is indicated between the DN3a and DN3b stages. This figure is modified form Aifnatis 2008 and Rothenberg 2008 [9],[11]

Temporal gene expression and cell surface phenotype in T-cell development

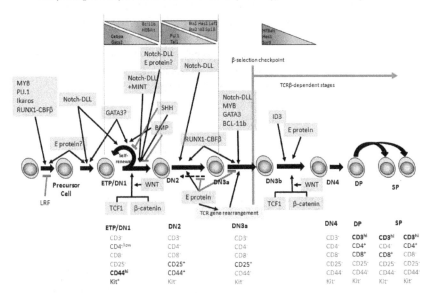

Figure 2. Regulatory factors in early T-cell development. The different stages of the cell differentiation are shown in the center starting with hematopoietic stem cells (HSC) and progressing to single positive cells. Above and below the line regulatory factors involved in the progression from one stage to another are indicated. Red lines indicated negatively active factors. The triangles at the top of the illustration indicate regulatory factors which are either upregulated or downregulated at indicated stages. For example, Tal1 expression decreases from the DN2 stage to the DN3a stage whereas Lef1 expression increased during that same transition. The solid blue line indicates the β-selection checkpoint with the long blue arrow indicating the TCRβ-dependent stages. At the bottom of the illustration the different cell surface phenotypes are shown below the corresponding stage in T-cell development. This figure is modified from Rothenberg 2008 [9].

3. Classifications

3.1. Recurring chromosomal aberrations

Chromosomal translocations which alter gene function were among the first clues to the genes and molecular mechanisms involved in abnormal T-cell biology. In T-ALL, approximately 50% of cases have cytogenetically detectable chromosomal abnormalities. There are at least two distinct molecular mechanisms of chromosomal translocations that can lead to abnormal T-cell biology (Figure 3). In one mechanism a strong regulatory element such as a promoter or enhancer is rearranged next to a gene resulting in abnormal expression of this gene. The affected gene typically encodes a transcription factor or a protein involved in cell cycle regulation. In the second mechanism the translocation results in a fusion protein. Frequently this fusion creates a novel protein that affects normal cell cycle regulation [16]. One of the hallmark features of T-ALL is translocations involving T-cell receptor genes, which are observed in majority of T-ALL patients. The bulk of these recurring aberrations involve strong transcriptional regulator elements from the T-cell receptor (TCR) genes being juxtaposed with genes encoding transcription factors. These alterations are frequently caused by erroneous V(D)J recombination events during T-cell development. Overall these chromosomal abnormalities lead to aberrant gene expression and proteins that alter normal growth, differentiation, and survival of T-cells and their precursors.

Two Mechanisms of aberrant gene activities by chromosomal translocations

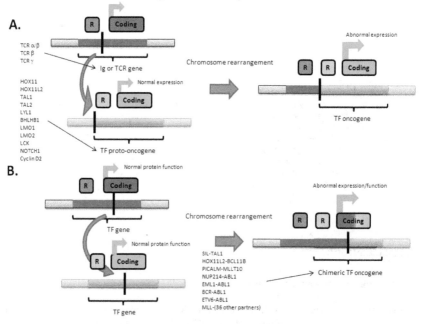

Figure 3. Two mechanisms of aberrant activities caused by chromosomal translocations. A. A strong promoter or enhancer is rearranged next to a proto-oncogene resulting in abnormal expression of the proto-oncogene. The TCR loci elements and recurring gene targets involved in T-cell leukemogenesis are indicated to the left. B. Chromosomal rearrangement between two transcription factors result in a chimeric transcription factor with oncogenic activity. Recurring gene fusions in T-cell leukemogenesis are indicated in the center below the arrow.

Approximately 35% of the observed cytogenetic abnormalities in T-ALL involve translocations that include the TCR alpha/delta chain at 14q11.2, the TCR beta chain at 7q34, and the TCR gamma chain at 7p14 (Table1). Among this group, rearrangements with the HOX11, HOX11L2, TAL1, TAL2, LYL1, BHLHB1, LMO1, LMO2, LCK, NOTCH1, and cyclin D2 genes are most frequently observed in patients [11]. Overexpression of LMO1, LMO2, or TAL1 is caused by rearrangements to the TCR delta chain in 3-9% of patients. About 3% of pediatric T-ALL is caused by ectopic TAL1(1p32) expression due to the t(1;14)(p32;q11) rearrangement [17]-[21]. Overexpression of HOX11(TLX1) is observed in greater than 30% of adult T-ALL when rearranged to the promoters of the TCR delta or TCR beta chains[22]. About 3-5% of patients have HOXA-TCR beta rearrangements. For example, the inv(7)(p15q34) and t(7;7)(p15;q34) rearrangement which results in up-regulation of the HOXA9, HOXA10 and HOXA11 genes [23],[24]. Rare translocations involving juxtaposition of the TCR gamma or the TCR alpha/delta chains to the LYL1 (19p13), TAL2 (9p32), or BHLH1(21q22) resulting in overexpression of these genes are also observed [25]-[28].

Several chromosomal translocations do not involve the TCR locus (Table1). In 10-25% of TAL1 positive T-ALL patients, TAL1 is expressed as result of an intrachromosomal deletion between the upstream ubiquitously expressed SIL gene as a result and TAL1 (SIL-TAL1)[29]-[31]. 20% of pediatric and 4% of adult cases of T-ALL have HOX11L2 (TLX3)-BCL11B fusion. This fusion causes ectopic expression of the HOX11L2/TLX3 gene [32],[33]. 8% of patients have the (10;11(p13;q14)/PICALM-MLLT10 rearrangement. In this case leukemogenesis is mediated through HOX gene upregulation via mistargeting of hDOT1l and H3K79 methylation [34],[35]. ABL1, a cytoplasmic tyrosine kinase, fusion genes have been identified in approximately 8% of T-ALL case. The NUP214-ABL1 fusion, which results in a constitutively active tyrosine kinase with oncogenic potential, occurs in 6% of both adult and children patients and is the most frequent ABL1 fusion gene observed. EMl1-ABL1, BCR-ABL1, and ETV6-ABL1 gene fusions are rarely observed in T-ALL but are frequent in other hematologic malignancies [36], [37]. ETV6, which is an important hematopoietic regulatory factor, fusion genes have been observed in both B-ALL (9.6%) and T-ALL patients (5%)[38],[39]. A significant cytogenetically visible deletion on chromosome 9p involves CDKN2A and CDKN2B genes, incidence of which varies from being rare to 70% in T-ALL cases [40]-[42]. In 5-10% of T-ALL patients, gene rearrangements involving MLL gene are observed. The MLL gene can fuse to at least 36 different translocation partner genes [43],[44]. Although there are a wide variety of chromosomal aberrations, the number of genes affected is relatively small. All of these genes are important for normal T-cell development.

3.2. Recurring genetic mutations

Several genes associated with T-ALL pathogenesis have mutations which are not cytogenetically visible. Some of the most frequently mutated genes are NOTCH1, FBXW7, PTEN, CDKN2A/B, CDKN1B, 6q15-16.1, PHF6, WT1, LEF1, JAK1, IL7R, FLT3, NRAS, BCL11B, and PTPN2 (Table2). Many of these genes were identified by gene expression profiling using microarrays or by whole genome sequencing analysis. Below some of these genes and their role in T-ALL is described briefly.

Recurring Translocations in T-ALL

TCR Rearrangements			Non-TCR Rerrangements		
Gene	Rearrangement	Frequency	Gene	Rearrangement	Frequency
TAL1	t(1;14) (p32;q11) t(1;7)(p32;q34)	~3 of T-ALL	TAL1	STIL-TAL1 (1p32 deletion)	12-25% T-ALL
TAL2	t(7;9)(q34;q32)	rare	HOXA	PICALM-MLLT10 (t(10;11) (p13;q14)) MLL-MLLT1 (t(11;19) (q23;p13)) SET-NUP214 9q34 deletions	
LMO1	t(11;14) (p15;q11) t(7;11) (q34;p15)	6-8% of T-ALL	ABL1	EML1-ABL1 (t(9:14) (q34;q32)) BCR-ABL1 (t(9;22)(q34;q11)) ETV6-ABl1 (t(9;12)(q34;p13)) NUP214-ABL1	8% T-ALL for ABL1 6% T-ALL for NUP214
LMO2	t(11;14) (p13;q11) t(7;11) (q34;p13) 11p13 deletions		ETV6	ETV6-JAK2 (t(9;12)(p24;p13) ETV6-ARNT (t(1;12)(q21;p13)	Rare
HOX11	t(10;14) (q24;q11) t(7;10) (q34;q24)	30% of T-ALL			
HOX11L2	t(5;14) (q35;q32)	20% Childhood T-ALL 4% Adult T-ALL			
HOXA	Inv(7)(p15q34) t(7;7)(p15;q34)				
LYL1	t(7;19) (q34;p13)	rare			

Table 1. Table of recurring translocation involved in T-ALL. The rearrangements are divided into those involving TCR and non-TCR loci.

Recurring genetic alterations in T-ALL		
Gene	Alteration	Frequency
Notch1	Sequence mutations	~50% of T-ALL
FBW7	Sequence mutations	~20% of T-ALL
PTEN	Deletions/Sequence mutations	6-8% of T-ALL
CDKN2A/B	Deletions	30-70% of T-ALL
CDKN1B	Deletions/Sequence mutations	12% of T-ALL
6q15-16.1	Deletions	12% of T-ALL
PHF6	Deletions/Sequence mutations	16% of childhood T-ALL 38% of adult T-ALL
WT1	Frameshift mutations	13% childhood T-ALL 12% of adult T-ALL
LEF1	Focal deletions/sequence mutations	15% of childhood T-ALL
JAK1	Sequence mutations	18% of adult T-ALL
IL7R	Gain of function mutation	9% of T-ALL
FLT3	Internal tandem duplication	4% of adult T-ALL 3% of childhood T-ALL
NRAS	Sequence mutations	10% childhood T-ALL
BCL11	Deletions/Sequence mutations	9% of all T-ALL case 16% of T-ALL cases with HOX11 overexpression
PTPN2	Deletion	6% of T-ALL

Table 2. Table indicating recurring genetic alterations in T-ALL. The type of alteration and frequency of occurrence in T-ALL cases is indicated.

3.2.1. Notch1 signaling pathway in T-ALL

Activating or loss of function NOTCH1 mutations are observed in ~34-71% of T-ALL and is one of the most significant T-ALL oncogene [45]-[49]. NOTCH is involved in the regulation of several cellular processes including differentiation, proliferation, apoptosis, adhesion, and spatial development [50],[51]. The importance of NOTCH1 in leukemogenesis was first discovered in a rare translocation t(7;9) that fuses the intracellular form of NOTCH1 to the TCR beta promoter and enhancer sequences. This rare fusion leads to a truncated and constitutively activated form of NOTCH1 termed TAN1 [52]. Other Notch isoforms also show oncogenic activity. Notch2 sequences were able to induce leukemogenesis in cats and overexpression of Notch3 in mice resulted in multi-organ infiltration by T lymphoblasts [53],[54]. The majority of T-ALL cases with active Notch1 arise due to mutations in the Notch1's heterodimerization (HD) domain and/or the PEST domain (proline-, glutamic-acid-, serine-, and threonine-rich domain)[46]. Mutations in the HD domain appear to make the NOTCH1 receptor susceptible to ligand-independent proteolysis and activation (Figure 4b), whereas, mutations in the PEST domain interfere with recognition of the intracellular form of NOTCH1 by the FBW7 ubiquitin ligase (Figure 4c) [45],[46],[55]-[62]. Notch1 is a single-transmembrane receptor with an extracellular, transmembrane, and intracellular subunits. Initially the cell-membrane-bound Notch protein is a single protein. After maturation when the protein is cleaved into two subunits the extracellular and intracellular subunits are linked non-covalently via the HD domains. On the extracellular domain multiple epidermal growth factor (EGF)-like repeats bind ligands namely, Delta-like ligand (DLL1), DLL2, DLL4, Jagged1 and Jagged 2. Ligand binding initiates two cleavage events by the ADAM family of metalloproteinases and the γ-secretase complex to release the intracellular form of NOTCH from the membrane. Two nuclear localization domains in NOTCH lead to its translocation to the nucleus [62]. Once in the nucleus, NOTCH associates with CSL (CBF1/suppressor of hairless/Lag1). Transcriptional activation of NOTCH-target genes begins once the NOTCH/CSL complex recruits the co-activator proteins like mastermind-like 1 and the histone acetyl transferase p300 (Figure 4a) [63]. The C-terminal domain of NOTCH contains the PEST domain. This domain is targeted for ubiquitination by FBW7 and subsequent proteasome-mediated degradation. Mutations in the PEST domain can increase the half-life of NOTCH protein resulting in aberrant activation of NOTCH-target genes [58],[59],[61]. Together, aberrant stabilization or activation of the intracellular form of NOTCH1 directly links to T-cell leukemogenesis.

Notch Signaling and mutations

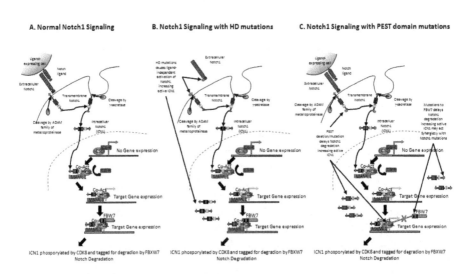

Figure 4. The Notch1 signaling pathway and mutations involved in aberrant Notch1 activation. A. Depiction of normal Notch1 signaling. Binding of Notch ligand to the extracellular Notch1 triggers a conformation change in the heterodi-merization domain (HD). This allows cleavage first by a metalloproteinase of the ADAM family and then by γ-secre-tase. These cleavages releases Notch1 from the membrane allowing it to translocate into the nuclease. Once in the nucleus, Notch1 associates with a transcriptional complex composed of CSL (CBF1/suppressor of hairless/lag1) and mastermind-like 1 (MAML1) to activate Notch1 target genes. Notch1 then becomes associated with FBW7 and is tag-ged for degradation following ubiquitination. B. Mutations in the HD domains (indicated by a red star) result in ligand independent cleavage allowing aberrant release of Notch1 from the membrane. C. Mutations in the PEST domain of Notch1 or mutations in FBW7 interfere with ubiquitination of Notch1. This allows accumulation of intracellular Notch1 by reducing its degradation. The figure is modified from Aifantis 2008 [11].

Because NOTCH1 plays a significant role in T-cell leukemogenesis, its regulation has been studied extensively. Nearly 40% of Notch-responsive genes are regulators of cell metabolism and protein biosynthesis [64]. c-MYC, a master regulator of multiple biosynthesis and metabolic pathways, is a direct transcriptional target of Notch1. Notch1 binding sites in the MYC promoter have been shown to be important for MYC expression in T-ALL [64]-[67]. Constitutively active Notch1 was shown to activate the NF-κB pathway [68], an important regulator of cell survival, cell cycle, cell adhesion and cell migration. This activation can occur by the direct transcriptional activation of Relb and Nfkb2 as well as via a Notch1 and IKK complex interaction. Another Notch1 target is PTEN (phosphatase and tension homologue). PTEN is negatively regulated by Notch1 through the activity of HES1 and MYC, resulting in the deregulation of the PI3K-AKT metabolic pathway [69]. Finally, Notch1 is also involved in the regulation of the NFAT signaling pathway, where it regulates the pathway by altering expression of calcineurin, a calcium-activated phosphatase [70]. Overall, these findings emphasize the role of Notch1 in inducing T-cell leukemogenesis through multiple cell signaling pathways capable of regulating cell survival, proliferation and metabolism.

As mentioned above, FBW7 (F-box and WD repeat domain containing 7), an E3 ubiquitin ligase located on chromosome 4q31.3, is observed to be mutated in T-ALL with a frequency ranging from 8.6% to 16% [59],[61],[71]. FBW7 is part of the SCF complex (SKP1-Cullin-1-F box protein complex), which can target MYC, JUN, cyclin E, and Notch1 for ubiquitination coupled proteosomal degradation [60]. The WD40 domain of FBW7 contains a degron-binding pocket domain. This domain recognizes phosphothreonine in the consensus sequence I/L/P-T-P-X-X-S/E of protein substrates. Roughly 20% of T-ALL patients have mutations in FBW7 that destroys the degron-binding pocket. Moreover, the degron sequence of Notch1 (LTPSPES) located in the distal portion of its PEST domain is found to be mutated in T-ALL, thus extending Notch1 half-life and altering downstream signaling cascades. Interestingly, T-ALL patients frequently have mutations in both the FBW7 degron binding pocket as well as in the Notch1 degron sequence (Figure 4c) [58],[59],[61]. These combined mutations elevate intracellular Notch1 activity and therefore, enhances leukemia manifestation. Current studies suggest FBW7 mutations induce T-cell leukemogenesis by disrupting Notch1 regulation.

PTEN (phosphatase and tensin homolog deleted on chromosome 10) is deleted or mutated in 6-8% of T-ALL cases. The major substrate of PTEN is PIP_3 (phosphatidylinositol-3,4,5-triphosphate). PTEN activity prevents the accumulation of PIP_3, thus limiting or terminating activation of a cascade of PI3K-dependent signaling molecules. The expression of PTEN has been shown to be negatively regulated by Notch1. PTEN appears to be required for optimal negative selection in the thymus. Loss of PTEN is characterized by overexpression of the c-myc oncogene and induction of lymphomagenesis within the thymus [69],[72]. Therefore PTEN appears to be an important tumor-suppressor involved in T-cell leukemogenesis.

3.2.2. Cell cycle, apoptosis, and transcription regulators in T-ALL

Deletions in CDKN2A and CDKN2B are significant secondary abnormities in pediatric T-ALL. Loss of the tumor suppressor CDKN2A/B expression is observed in 30-70% of T-ALL cases and can occur due to chromosomal translocation, promoter hypermethylation, somatic mutation, or gene deletions [40],[42]. CDKN2A and CDKN2B are located adjacent on chromosome 9p21. CDKN2A encodes p16[INK4a](cyclin-dependent kinase inhibitor)/p14[ARF]while CDKN2B encodes p15[INKb]. These genes block cell division during the G_1/S phase of the cell cycle by inhibiting cyclin/CDK-4/6 complexes [73],[74]. The principle mode of CDKN2A inactivation occurs via genomic deletions which can usually be detected by FISH [41]. Loss of function of CDKN1B (cyclin-dependent kinase inhibitor 1B) gene, located on 12p13.2, have been observed in 12% of T-ALL cases [75]. Similar to CDKN2A and CDKN2B, CDKN1B acts as a tumor suppressor. Inactivation of CDKN1B leads to overexpression of D-cyclins, thereby inhibiting the cells ability to maintain quiescence in G0. Therefore, CDKN2/B and CDKN1B play an important role in abnormal T-cell biology by regulating cell cycle progression.

12% of pediatric T-ALL cases have deletion in 6q15-16.1 [75]. The single most down regulated gene in this region is caspase 8 associated protein 2 (CASP8AP2). Deletion of CASP8AP2 probably interferes with Fas-mediated apoptosis. In gene expression profiling study, loss of CASP8AP2 was not observed in any pre-B-ALL samples [75], indicating deletions to 6q15-16.1 maybe a hallmark of T-ALL.

The X-linked plant homeodomain (PHD) finger 6 (PHF6) gene has inactivating mutations in 16% of pediatric and 38% of adult primary T-ALL cases [76]. Mutations in PHF6 are limited to male T-ALL cases. Consequently, this gene may be responsible for the increased incidence of T-ALL cases in males. Loss of expression of the PHF6 gene was associated with leukemia driven by abnormal expression of the homeobox transcription factor oncogenes. PHF6 gene encodes a protein with two plant homeodomain-like zinc finger domains. A recent study demonstrated that PHF6 copurifies with the nucleosome remodeling and deacetylation (NuRD) complex, implicating its role in chromatin regulation [77].

The WT1 (Wilms tumor) tumor suppressor gene is mutated in 13.2% of pediatric and 11.7% of adult T-ALL cases [78],[79]. The WT1 is known to be a transcriptional activator of the erythropoietin gene. Loss of WT1 expression results in diminished erythropoietin receptor (EpoR) expression in hematopoietic progenitors, suggesting that activation of the EpoR gene by Wt1 is an important mechanism in normal hematopoiesis [80]. WT1 mutations are frequently prevalent in T-ALL cases harboring chromosomal rearrangements associated with abnormal expression of the homeobox transcription oncogenes, HOX11, HOX11L2, and HOXA9 [79]. This suggests that the recurrent genetic mutations in WT1 are associated with abnormal HOX gene expression in T-ALL period

Lymphoid enhance factor 1 (LEF1) gene is mutated in 15% of pediatric T-ALL cases [81]. Inactivation of LEF1 was associated with increased expression of MYC and MYC targets, a gene expression signature consistent with developmental arrest at a cortical stage of T-cell differentiation. Interestingly, T-ALL cases with LEF1 mutation lacked overexpression of TAL1, HOX11, HOX11L2 and HOXA genes suggesting that LEF1 acts via different molecular pathways in T-cell leukemogenesis. In fact, The LEF family of DNA-binding transcription factors interacts with nuclear β-catenin in the WNT signaling pathway. The loss of LEF1 may result in the relief of transcriptional repression of MYC in T-ALL cases. It was reported that LEF1 probably contributes to T-ALL pathogenesis by acting in concert with NOTCH1 to promote up-regulation of MYC expression. In this case LEF1 also relieves transcriptional repression of MYC to allow its maximum overexpression by Notch1 [81].

3.2.3. JAK/STAT signaling pathway in T-ALL

About 18% of adult and 2% of pediatric T-ALL cases have activating mutations in the Janus Kinase 1 (JAK1) [38]. The JAK family (JAK1, JAK2, JAK3, and TYK2) function as signal transducers to control cell proliferation, survival, and differentiation. They are nonreceptor tyrosine kinases that associate with cytokine receptors to phosphorylate tyrosine residues of the target proteins. This process regulates the recruitment and activation of STAT proteins. The JAK/STAT signaling cascade is an important regulator of normal T-cell development. Each JAK family member associates with a different subset of cytokine receptors. JAK1 regulates the class II cytokine receptors as well as receptors that use the gp130 or γ_c receptor subunit. These class of cytokine receptors are involved in controlling lymphoid development [82],[83]. The majority of the JAK1 kinase mutations observed in T-ALL cases result in unregulated tyrosine kinase activity. T-ALL cases with mutations in JAK1 appear to be associated with different T-ALL subgroups than patients harboring aberrant expressions of the homeobox transcription factors HOX11 and HOX11L2 [38]. JAK1 is involved in the regulation of both interleukin 7 receptor (IL7R) and protein tyrosine phosphatase non-receptor type 2 (PTPN2) [84],[85].

The interleukin 7 receptor (IL7R) has a gain-of-function mutation in exon 6 in 9% of T-ALL cases [85]. Several lines of evidence suggest IL7R plays an important role in T-cell leukemogenesis. IL-7 and IL7R signaling are essential for normal T-cell development. Deficiency of IL-7 and IL7R in mice caused reduction of non-functional T cells and showed an early block in thymocyte development [86]-[89]. Loss of IL7R function also results in severe combined immunodeficiency in humans [90]. Increased expression of IL7R was associated with spontaneous thymic lymphomas in mice. Furthermore, Notch1 has been shown to transcriptionally upregulate IL7R receptor gene [91]. Mutations in exon 6 of IL7R promotes de novo formation of intermolecular disulfide bonds between IL7R mutant subunits, which triggers constitutive activation of tyrosine kinase JAK1 regardless of regulation by IL-7, $\gamma_{c,}$ or JAK3. Gene expression profiles for IL7R mutations are generally associated with the T-ALL subgroup harboring HOX11L2 rearrangements and HOXA deregulation [85].

Inactivation of protein tyrosine phosphatase non-receptor type 2 (PTPN2) gene is observed in ~6% of T-ALL cases [84],[92]. PTPN2 encodes a tyrosine phosphatase, located on chromosome 18p11.3-11.2, that negatively regulates JAK/STAT pathway and NUP214-ABL1 kinase activity. Loss of PTPN2 results in activation of the JAK/STAT pathway and increased T-cell proliferation by cytokines. Unlike JAK1 mutations, deletions in PTPN2 gene appear to be restricted to T-ALL cases which specifically overexpress HOX11 [84]. Therefore mutations in PTPN2 probably play a role in T-cell leukemogenesis by deregulating tyrosine kinase signaling.

Activating mutations in the FMS-like tyrosine kinase 3 (FLT3) gene are amongst the most common genetic aberrations in acute myeloid leukemia [93]-[95]. In T-ALL, FLT3 mutations are relatively rare with a frequency of approximately 4% in adult and 3% in pediatric cases. [96]-[98]. FLT3 encodes a class III membrane tyrosine kinase that is expressed in early hematopoietic stem cells. Normally FLT3 is activated when bound by the FLT3 ligand (FL). This interaction causes receptor dimerization and kinase activity resulting in activation of downstream signaling pathways such as Ras/MAP kinase, PIK3/AKT, and STAT5. The most frequent FLT3 mutation involves a duplication of the juxtamembrane (JM) domain. This mutation leads to dimerization of FLT3 in the absence of FLT3 ligand (FL), autophosphorylation of the receptor and constitutive activation of the tyrosine kinase domain, which triggers uncontrolled proliferation and resistance to apoptotic signaling though activation of the PIK3/AKT, Ras/ MAPK and JAK2/STAT pathways [98]-[100].

The B-cell chronic lymphocytic leukemia (CLL)/lymphoma 11B (BCL11B) gene has mutations in 16% of T-ALL patients with HOX11 overexpression. However, in unselected patients, deletions or missense mutations for BCL11B were observed in only 9% of cases. This suggests that BCL11 mutations probably occur across all subtypes of T-ALL [101]. BCL11B is located on human chromosome 14q32.2 and encodes a kruppel-like C_2H_2 zinc finger protein which acts as a transcriptional repressor. Loss of function mutations in BCL11B gene in mice leads to developmental arrest of T-cell in DN2-DN3 stage, acquisition of NK-like features, and aberrant self-renewal activity. Transcriptional activation of IL-2 expression in activated T-cell is mediated by BCL11B via its interaction with p300 co-activator at the IL-2 promoter [102]-[106]. Because of BCL11B's role in normal T-cell development, it plays an important role in T-cell leukemogenesis.

Approximately 10% of childhood T-ALL cases have mutations in NRAS oncogene located on chromosome 1p13.2, which is involved in the malignant transformation of many cells [107]. The recurrence of NRAS mutations in T-ALL cases suggests that NRAS is involved in abnormal T-cell biology.

3.3. Gene expression profiles

Whole genome sequencing and gene expression profiles provide a more comprehensive view of the genetic alterations involved in T-cell leukemia. A recent microarray-based gene expression study classified T-ALL cases into major subgroups corresponding to leukemic arrest at different stages of thymocyte differentiation. Currently there are 3 subtypes of T-ALL cases which include the HOXA/MEISI, TLX1/3 and TAL1-overexpressing subtype [108], the LEF1-inactivated subtype [81], and the early T-cell precursor phenotype [109] (Figure 5). Leukemic arrest at early pro-T thymocytes (DN2 cells) were characterized by high levels of expression of the LYL1 gene. Arrest in early cortical thymocytes (DN3 cells) were characterized by changes in HOX11/TLX1 expression. Arrest in late cortial thymocytes (DP cells) were characterized by changes in the TAL1/LMO1 expression. Aberrant HOX11L2/TLX3 activation was also identified as being involved in T cell leukemogenesis (Figure 4) [108]. TAL1 and LYL1 are members of the basic helix-loop-helix (bHLH) family of transcription factors, LMO1 is member of the LIM-only domain genes (LMO), and HOX11 and HOX11L2 belongs to the homeobox gene family.

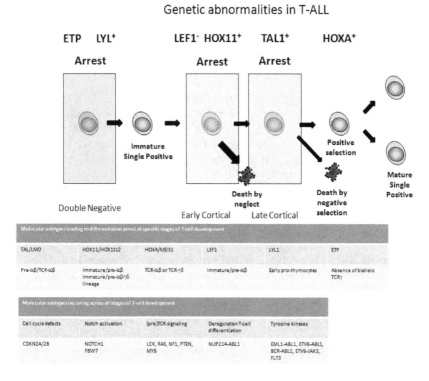

Figure 5. Gene subtypes resulting in differentiation arrest at specific stages of T-cell development. The illustration shows the progression of T-cell development from the double negative stages to the mature single positive stage. The colored rectangles indicates stages of leukemic arrest. Overexpression of LYL, HOX11, TAL1, and HOXA lead to differentiation arrest at the double negative stage, early cortical stage, late cortical stage, and positive selections stage, respectively. Loss of Lef1 expression results in early cortical leukemic arrest. The table below indicates the molecular subtypes leading to differentiation arrest at specific stages of T-cell development and the molecular subtypes occurring across all the stages of T-cell development.

Recently whole genome sequencing of early T-cell precursor acute lymphoblastic leukemia (ETP-ALL) identified several genes involved in abnormal T-cell biology [10]. 15% of T-ALL cases are ETP-ALL. Phenotypically ETP-ALL is negative for the cell surface markers CD1a and CD8, has little to no expression of CD5, and has aberrant expression of myeloid and hematopoietic stem cell markers. This study performed whole genome sequencing on 12 children with ETP-ALL. The frequency of the mutations identified from these 12 cases was then accessed in 94 cases of T-ALL. Of these 94 cases 52 cases had ETP and 42 had a non-ETP pediatric T-ALL. Even though an average of 1140 sequence mutations and 12 structural variations in the genome were identified per ETP case, they were able to narrow down the number of affected genes to 3 group and 3 novel genes (DNM2, ECT2L, and RELN). 67% of the cases were characterized by activating mutations in genes involved in the regulation of cytokine receptor and RAS signaling. These genes included NRAS, KRAS, FLT3, IL7R, JAK3, JAK1, SH2B3 and BRAF. 58% of the cases were characterized by inactivating lesions that disrupted hematopoietic development. These genes included GATA3, ETV6, RUNX1, IKZF1, and EP300. 48% of the cases were characterized by changes in histone modifying genes (EZH2, EED, SUZ12, SETD2, and EP300) [10]. From gene expression profiling and whole genome sequencing we are beginning to obtain a more complete picture of the genes involved in abnormal T-cell biology.

MicroRNA expression profiling found 10 detectable miRNAs in human T-ALL cells, five of these miRNAs (miR-19b, miR-20a, miR-26a, miR-92, and miR223) were predicted to target tumor suppressors genes implicated in T-ALL [110]. These five miRNA's were able to accelerate leukemia development in a mouse model. Furthermore, it was shown that these five miRNAs produced overlapping and cooperative effects of the tumor suppressor genes IKAROS, PTEN, BIM, PHF6, NF1 and FBXW7 in T-ALL pathogenesis. miR223 appears to be the most overexpressed miRNA in leukemia. These results indicate the important role that miRNA's play in abnormal T-cell biology.

3.4. Basic helix-loop-helix proteins

As mentioned early, some of the most common recurrent chromosomal aberrations in abnormal T-cell biology involved chromosomal translocations of the TCR gene to the basic helix-loop-helix (bHLH) genes (MYC, TAL1, TAL2, LYL1, bHLHB1), the cysteine-rich (LIM-domain) genes (LMO1, LMO2), or the homeodomain genes (HOX11/TLX1), HOX11L2/TLX3, members of the HOXA cluster) (Table1). The most common bHLH gene with aberrant expression observed in T-ALL cases is the transcriptional regulator TAL1 (T-cell acute lymphocytic leukemia 1; also known as SCL). It was first identified in T-ALL patients with the t(1;14)(p32;q11) translocation [17],[18],[20],[21]. This chromosomal rearrangement, which is observed in 3% of cases, causes ectopic TAL1 expression by placing TAL1 under control of the TCRδ oncogene [19]-[21],[111]. 12%-25% of T-ALL cases have a submicroscopic 90-kb deletion that fuses the TAL1 coding sequence to the first exon of the SIL gene (SCL interrupting locus). This rearrangement leads to dysregulation of TAL1 expression [17],[29]-[31]. The majority of T-ALL cases, up to 60%, show ectopic TAL1 expression with no detectable TAL1 gene rearrangements [112]. Gene expression profiling has shown that ectopic expression of TAL1 results in leukemic arrest in late cortical thymocytes (Figure 5) [108]. These results show that activation of TAL1 gene is required for the leukemic phenotype of T-cells.

The TAL1 gene, located on chromosome 1p32, encodes a class II basic helix-loop-helix factor [113]. The protein binds DNA as a heterodimer with the ubiquitously expressed class I bHLH genes known as E-proteins such as E2A or HEB. These heterodimers recognize an E box sequence (CANNTG)[114]. TAL1 positively and negatively modulates transcription of targets gene as a large complex consisting of an E-protein, the LIM-only proteins LMO1/2, GATA1/2, Ldb1, and other associated coregulators. This complex usually binds a composite DNA elements containing an E box and a GATA-binding site separated by 9 or 10 bp (Figure 6) [115]-[117]. It was shown recently that in T-ALL cells TAL1, GATA-3, LMO1, and RUNX1 together form a core transcription regulatory circuit to reinforce and stabilize the TAL1-directed leukemogenic program [118].

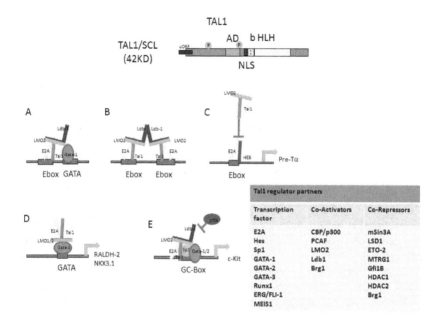

Figure 6. Model of TAL1 complexs and target sites. A. TAL1 complex binding to an E-box and GATA box. B. TAL1 complex binding to a double E-box. C. TAL1 complex binding to a single E-box. D. TAL1 complex binding to a single GATA site showing activation of either the RALDH-2 or NKX3.1 genes. E. TAL1 complex binding to a GC-box with activation of c-kit. The table to the lower right shows the different TAL1 regulator partners. The partners are divided into three categories transcription factors, co-activators, or co-repressors.

TAL1 expression is essential for hematopoiesis. It is required for specification of hematopoietic stem cells during embryonic development and it is necessary for erythroid maturation. Normal expression of TAL1 is restricted to the DN1-DN2 subset of immature CD4-/CD8- thymocytes with ectopic expression resulting in leukemic arrest in late cortical thymocytes [108].

Two models have been proposed for TAL1-induced leukemogenesis. In the prevailing model TAL1 acts as a transcriptional repressor by blocking the transcriptional activities of E2A, HEB, and/or E2-2 through its heterodimerization with these E-proteins. TAL1 may mediate its inhibitory effect by interfering with E2A-mediated recruitment of chromatin-remodeling complex which activate transcription [114],[119]-[121]. It also been shown to associate with several corepressors including HDAC1, HDAC2, mSin3A, Brg1, LSD1, ETO-2, Mtgr1, and Gfi1-b (Figure 6) [122]. In human T-ALL TAL1 transcriptional repression may be mediated by TAL1-E2A DNA binding and recruitment of the corepressors LSD1 and/or HP1-α [123]. In the other model TAL1 induces leukemogenesis through inappropriate gene activation [124]. At least two genes RALDH2 and NKX3.1 are transcriptionally activated by TAL1 and GATA-3 dependent recruitment of the TAL1-LMO-Ldb1 complex [125],[126]. As a transcriptional activator TAL1 has been shown to associate with the coactivators p300 and P/CAF (Figure 6) [127],[128]. Both of these complexes contain HAT activities. The prevalence of histone-modifying enzymes in TAL1 complexes suggests that one function of TAL1 is to regulate chromatin states of its target genes.

TAL1 and the lymphoblastic leukemia-derived sequence 1 (LYL1) share 90% sequence identity in their bHLH motif [26]. Like TAL1, LYL1 role in leukemogenesis was discovered by studying chromosomal rearrangements. It is expressed by adult hematopoietic cells and is overexpressed in T-ALL. Gene expression profiling showed that overexpression of LYL1 resulted in leukemic arrest at pro T-cell (Double negative) stage of T-cell differentiation (Figure 5) [108]. In mouse embryos LYL1 and TAL1 expression overlaps in hematopoietic development, developing vasculature and endocardium. At the molecular level LYL1 controls expression of several genes involved in the maturation and stabilization of the newly formed blood vessels [129]. Therefore, bHLH proteins play an important role in abnormal T-cell biology.

3.5. LIM domain proteins

Aberrant expression of the LMO1 and LMO2 proteins is observed in 45% of T-ALL cases. The discovery of the LMO1 and LMO2 genes adjacent to the chromosomal translocations t(11;14) (p15q11) and t(11;14)(p13;q11) was the first indication that these proteins were involved in T-cell leukemogenesis [130]-[132]. The LMO family (LMO1, LMO2, LMO3, and LMO4) encodes genes that have two cysteine-rich zinc coordinating LIM domains. The LIM domain is found in a variety of proteins including the homeodomain-containing transcription factors, kinases, and adaptors. Despite the presence of 2 zinc finger motifs, LMO1 and LMO2 genes do not appear to bind DNA. Instead the LMO proteins probably act as scaffolding protein to form multiprotein complex through their interaction with the LIM domain binding protein 1 (LDB1) (Figure 6) [116].

Leukemogenesis by aberrant expression of LMO1 or LMO2 is thought to occur via two mechanisms. In the first mechanism aberrant expression or abnormal LMO proteins forms a dysfunctional multiprotein complexes that alters the expression of the target genes by directly binding to their promoters [133]-[136]. In the second mechanism abnormal LMO1 or LMO2 complexes displace the LMO4 complex. This results in arrest of T-cell development at the DP stage [137].

LMO2 function is necessary for normal T-cell development. In fact, LMO2 has been shown to interact with several factors involved in aberrant T-cell biology. As mentioned above TAL1 may regulate its target genes through the TAL1-LMO-Ldb1 complex (Figure 6). Ectopic expression of LMO1 and LMO2 leads to accumulation of immature DN T cells in mice with subsequent leukemia manifestation with a long latency, suggesting the role of LMO is important for the development of tumors but is not self-sufficient [26],[138],[139]. Ectopic expression of both TAL1 and LMO1 in mice accelerated the progression to leukemogenesis (Figure 7). In this case thymic expression of the TAL1 and LMO1 oncogenes induced expansion of the ETP/DN1 to DN4 population and lead to T-ALL in ~120 days. The acquisition of a Notch1 gain-of-function mutation was proposed to be the rationale behind this increase in leukemia penetrance. In fact, thymic expression of all three oncogenes Notch1, TAL1 and LMO1 induced T-ALL with high penetrance in 31 days, the time necessary for clonal expansion (Figure 7) [140]. These studies suggest that aberrant LMO proteins are key players in abnormal T-cell biology.

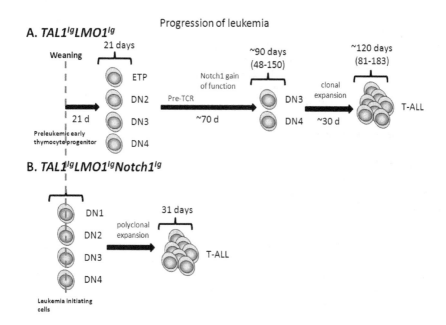

Figure 7. Model of progression to leukemia via TAL1, LMO1 and Notch1. The dashed line indicates the time of wean-ing. The number of days to differentiation arrest and finally T-ALL are shown above the cell stages. A. Shows the num-bers of days to full T-ALL in mice with TAL1 and LMO1 oncogenes. Note the 70 day delay for a Notch1 gain of function mutation. B. Shows the number of days to full T-ALL in mice with TAL1, LMO1, and Notch1 oncogenes. Note the delay is ~30 days the time necessary for clonal expansion. This figure is modified from Tremblay et al 2010 [140].

3.6. Homeobox genes

Dysregulated expression of HOX-type transcription factors occurs in 30-40% of T-ALL cases [23],[24],[32]. The HOX genes play an important role in hematopoiesis [141]. The majority of the HOXA, HOXB and HOXC genes clusters are expressed in hematopoietic stem cells and immature progenitor compartments. Furthermore, these genes are down regulated during differentiation and maturation of hematopoiesis [142],[143]. In T-ALL dysregulation of the HOXA gene cluster is a frequent recurring aberration. Upregulation of HOXA9, HOXA10, and HOXA11 occurs in T-ALL cases when the TCR beta regulatory elements are juxtaposed with these genes [16].

Two orphan HOX proteins (HOX11 and HOX11L2) have been implicated in T-cell leukemogen-esis [144]. Overexpression of HOX11 is observed in 30% of T-ALL cases because of two recurring translocation events. This gene is also frequently overexpressed in T-ALL cases in the ab-sence of genetic rearrangements. Mice deficient in HOX11 fail to develop a spleen, implicat-ing its role in spleen organogenesis [145]. Normally HOX11 is not expressed in thymocytes. Ectopic expression of HOX11 in T-cells caused a block at the DP stage of T-cell differentiation (Figure 5). This is consistent with genetic profiling studies which showed that overexpression of HOX11 results in leukemic arrest at early cortical thymocytes stage (Figure 5) [108]. Overexpression of HOX11 in hematopoietic stems cells of mice developed T-cell leukemia. However, the long latency of tumorigenesis suggests other genetic abnormalities are required [146]-[148]. It should be noted that nearly all HOX11 T-ALL cases have activating NOTCH1 mutation. It has been proposed that HOX11 binding to the Groucho-related TLE corepressor was necessary for maximal transcriptional regulation of Notch1-responsive genes. This suggests that HOX11 and Notch1 may synergistically regulate transcription in T-ALL [149].

3.7. Epigenetic modifications

Aberrant changes in DNA methylation and histone modifications occur frequently in all cancers. Estimates vary but studies suggest that there are approximately 100 epigenetic changes for every DNA based genetic mutation. Consequently epigenetic modifications will almost certainly play an important role in T-cell leukemogenesis.

Comparative genomic hybridization data of T-ALL primary samples has shown recurrent deletions in 25% of T-ALL cases in EZH2 and SUZ12 genes. These genes are members of the polycomb repressor complex 2 (PRC2) and involved in establishing the repressive H3K27me3 mark. Activation of Notch1 was shown to cause the loss of the H3K27me3 mark by antagonizing the activity of PRC2. This data implicates histone modifications and PRC2 as important regulatory factors in T-cell leukemogenesis [150].

The CpG island methylator phenotype (CIMP) has been used to characterize T-ALL patients. The CIMP+ phenotype has a large number of hypermethylated genes with the CIMP- having a low number of hypermethylated genes. Analysis of the methylation status of 20 genes, the majority of which are implicated in abnormal T-cell biology, in 61 pediatric T-ALL patients and 11 healthy children showed a difference in the CIMP pattern. On average patients had 2.4 hypermethylated loci where none of the normal individual's loci where hypermethylated [151]. Therefore changes in the patterns of CpG island methylation at critical genes can be associated with specific tumorigenesis and consequently may be playing an important role in T-cell leukemogenesis.

4. Summary

Although there are a large number of genes involved in the molecular morphogenesis of T-cell leukemogenesis, many of the genes act through related pathways. This has helped us clarify the different genetic subtypes of T-ALL improving our risk stratification of T-ALL. Furthermore understanding the different genetic subtypes is allowing for personalized chemotherapy. Powerful new tools such as next-generation sequencing aid in identifying more relevant recurring lesions in leukemogenesis. This is resulting in the development of better therapeutic agents and methods. Because of improved supportive care, better risk stratification and personalized chemotherapy the 5-year survival of pediatric acute lymphoblastic leukemia has increase to 85% [152]. Even though we have made significant progress in the understanding of the molecular morphogenesis of T-ALL there are still significant gaps in our knowledge of the genes involved in leukemogenesis.

Acknowledgements

We are grateful to members of the Huang laboratory for their suggestions and comments. We also apologize to those whose work could not be cited due to space constraints. This work was supported by grants from the National Institute of Health (R01 HL090589 and R01 HL091929 to SH; 5T32CA9126-34 to BP: R01HL095674 to YQ).

Author details

Michael Litt[1], Bhavita Patel[2], Ying Li[2], Yi Qiu[3,4] and Suming Huang[1,3]

1 Medical Education Center, Ball State University, Muncie, IN, USA

2 Department of Bichemistry and Molecular Biology, University of Florida, College of Medicine, Gainesville, FL, USA

3 Shands Cancer Center, University of Florida, College of Medicine, Gainesville, FL, USA

4 Anatomy and Cell Biology, University of Florida, College of Medicine, Gainesville, FL, USA

References

[1] Pui CH, Relling MV, Downing JR. Acute lymphoblastic leukemia. *N Engl J Med.* 2004;350(15):1535-1548. Prepublished on 2004/04/09 as DOI 10.1056/NEJMra023001.

[2] van Grotel M, Meijerink JP, Beverloo HB, et al. The outcome of molecular-cytogenetic subgroups in pediatric T-cell acute lymphoblastic leukemia: a retrospective study of patients treated according to DCOG or COALL protocols. *Haematologica.* 2006;91(9): 1212-1221. Prepublished on 2006/09/08 as DOI.

[3] Iacobucci I, Papayannidis C, Lonetti A, Ferrari A, Baccarani M, Martinelli G. Cytogenetic and molecular predictors of outcome in acute lymphocytic leukemia: recent developments. *Curr Hematol Malig Rep.* 2012;7(2):133-143. Prepublished on 2012/04/25 as DOI 10.1007/s11899-012-0122-5.

[4] Kraszewska MD, Dawidowska M, Szczepanski T, Witt M. T-cell acute lymphoblastic leukaemia: recent molecular biology findings. *Br J Haematol.* 2012;156(3):303-315. Prepublished on 2011/12/08 as DOI 10.1111/j.1365-2141.2011.08957.x.

[5]   Akashi K, Reya T, Dalma-Weiszhausz D, Weissman IL. Lymphoid precursors. *Curr Opin Immunol*. 2000;12(2):144-150. Prepublished on 2000/03/14 as DOI.

[6]   Blom B, Spits H. Development of human lymphoid cells. *Annu Rev Immunol*. 2006;24:287-320. Prepublished on 2006/03/23 as DOI 10.1146/annurev.immunol. 24.021605.090612.

[7]   Boehm T, Bleul CC. Thymus-homing precursors and the thymic microenvironment. *Trends Immunol*. 2006;27(10):477-484. Prepublished on 2006/08/22 as DOI 10.1016/j.it. 2006.08.004.

[8]   Scimone ML, Aifantis I, Apostolou I, von Boehmer H, von Andrian UH. A multistep adhesion cascade for lymphoid progenitor cell homing to the thymus. *Proc Natl Acad Sci U S A*. 2006;103(18):7006-7011. Prepublished on 2006/04/28 as DOI 10.1073/pnas. 0602024103.

[9]   Rothenberg EV, Moore JE, Yui MA. Launching the T-cell-lineage developmental programme. *Nat Rev Immunol*. 2008;8(1):9-21. Prepublished on 2007/12/22 as DOI 10.1038/nri2232.

[10]   Zhang J, Ding L, Holmfeldt L, et al. The genetic basis of early T-cell precursor acute lymphoblastic leukaemia. *Nature*. 2012;481(7380):157-163. Prepublished on 2012/01/13 as DOI 10.1038/nature10725.

[11]   Aifantis I, Raetz E, Buonamici S. Molecular pathogenesis of T-cell leukaemia and lymphoma. *Nat Rev Immunol*. 2008;8(5):380-390. Prepublished on 2008/04/19 as DOI 10.1038/nri2304.

[12]   Naito T, Tanaka H, Naoe Y, Taniuchi I. Transcriptional control of T-cell development. *Int Immunol*. 2011;23(11):661-668. Prepublished on 2011/09/29 as DOI 10.1093/intimm/ dxr078.

[13]   von Boehmer H, Aifantis I, Gounari F, et al. Thymic selection revisited: how essential is it? *Immunol Rev*. 2003;191:62-78. Prepublished on 2003/03/05 as DOI.

[14]   Di Santo JP, Radtke F, Rodewald HR. To be or not to be a pro-T? *Curr Opin Immunol*. 2000;12(2):159-165. Prepublished on 2000/03/14 as DOI.

[15]   El Andaloussi A, Graves S, Meng F, Mandal M, Mashayekhi M, Aifantis I. Hedgehog signaling controls thymocyte progenitor homeostasis and differentiation in the thymus. *Nat Immunol*. 2006;7(4):418-426. Prepublished on 2006/03/07 as DOI 10.1038/ ni1313.

[16]   Look AT. Oncogenic transcription factors in the human acute leukemias. *Science*. 1997;278(5340):1059-1064. Prepublished on 1997/11/14 as DOI.

[17]   Aplan PD, Lombardi DP, Ginsberg AM, Cossman J, Bertness VL, Kirsch IR. Disruption of the human SCL locus by "illegitimate" V-(D)-J recombinase activity. *Science*. 1990;250(4986):1426-1429. Prepublished on 1990/12/07 as DOI.

[18] Begley CG, Aplan PD, Davey MP, et al. Demonstration of delta rec-pseudo J alpha rearrangement with deletion of the delta locus in a human stem-cell leukemia. *J Exp Med*. 1989;170(1):339-342. Prepublished on 1989/07/01 as DOI.

[19] Carroll AJ, Crist WM, Link MP, et al. The t(1;14)(p34;q11) is nonrandom and restricted to T-cell acute lymphoblastic leukemia: a Pediatric Oncology Group study. *Blood*. 1990;76(6):1220-1224. Prepublished on 1990/09/15 as DOI.

[20] Chen Q, Cheng JT, Tasi LH, et al. The tal gene undergoes chromosome translocation in T cell leukemia and potentially encodes a helix-loop-helix protein. *EMBO J*. 1990;9(2): 415-424. Prepublished on 1990/02/01 as DOI.

[21] Finger LR, Kagan J, Christopher G, et al. Involvement of the TCL5 gene on human chromosome 1 in T-cell leukemia and melanoma. *Proc Natl Acad Sci U S A*. 1989;86(13): 5039-5043. Prepublished on 1989/07/01 as DOI.

[22] Bergeron J, Clappier E, Radford I, et al. Prognostic and oncogenic relevance of TLX1/ HOX11 expression level in T-ALLs. *Blood*. 2007;110(7):2324-2330. Prepublished on 2007/07/05 as DOI 10.1182/blood-2007-04-079988.

[23] Soulier J, Clappier E, Cayuela JM, et al. HOXA genes are included in genetic and biologic networks defining human acute T-cell leukemia (T-ALL). *Blood*. 2005;106(1): 274-286. Prepublished on 2005/03/19 as DOI 10.1182/blood-2004-10-3900.

[24] Speleman F, Cauwelier B, Dastugue N, et al. A new recurrent inversion, inv(7)(p15q34), leads to transcriptional activation of HOXA10 and HOXA11 in a subset of T-cell acute lymphoblastic leukemias. *Leukemia*. 2005;19(3):358-366. Prepublished on 2005/01/28 as DOI 10.1038/sj.leu.2403657.

[25] Graux C, Cools J, Michaux L, Vandenberghe P, Hagemeijer A. Cytogenetics and molecular genetics of T-cell acute lymphoblastic leukemia: from thymocyte to lymphoblast. *Leukemia*. 2006;20(9):1496-1510. Prepublished on 2006/07/11 as DOI 10.1038/ sj.leu.2404302.

[26] Mellentin JD, Smith SD, Cleary ML. lyl-1, a novel gene altered by chromosomal translocation in T cell leukemia, codes for a protein with a helix-loop-helix DNA binding motif. *Cell*. 1989;58(1):77-83. Prepublished on 1989/07/14 as DOI.

[27] Wang J, Jani-Sait SN, Escalon EA, et al. The t(14;21)(q11.2;q22) chromosomal translocation associated with T-cell acute lymphoblastic leukemia activates the BHLHB1 gene. *Proc Natl Acad Sci U S A*. 2000;97(7):3497-3502. Prepublished on 2000/03/29 as DOI.

[28] Xia Y, Brown L, Yang CY, et al. TAL2, a helix-loop-helix gene activated by the (7;9) (q34;q32) translocation in human T-cell leukemia. *Proc Natl Acad Sci U S A*. 1991;88(24): 11416-11420. Prepublished on 1991/12/25 as DOI.

[29] Bash RO, Crist WM, Shuster JJ, et al. Clinical features and outcome of T-cell acute lymphoblastic leukemia in childhood with respect to alterations at the TAL1 locus: a Pediatric Oncology Group study. *Blood*. 1993;81(8):2110-2117. Prepublished on 1993/04/15 as DOI.

[30] Breit TM, Mol EJ, Wolvers-Tettero IL, Ludwig WD, van Wering ER, van Dongen JJ. Site-specific deletions involving the tal-1 and sil genes are restricted to cells of the T cell receptor alpha/beta lineage: T cell receptor delta gene deletion mechanism affects multiple genes. *J Exp Med*. 1993;177(4):965-977. Prepublished on 1993/04/01 as DOI.

[31] Brown L, Cheng JT, Chen Q, et al. Site-specific recombination of the tal-1 gene is a common occurrence in human T cell leukemia. *EMBO J*. 1990;9(10):3343-3351. Prepublished on 1990/10/01 as DOI.

[32] Bernard OA, Busson-LeConiat M, Ballerini P, et al. A new recurrent and specific cryptic translocation, t(5;14)(q35;q32), is associated with expression of the Hox11L2 gene in T acute lymphoblastic leukemia. *Leukemia*. 2001;15(10):1495-1504. Prepublished on 2001/10/06 as DOI.

[33] Su XY, Della-Valle V, Andre-Schmutz I, et al. HOX11L2/TLX3 is transcriptionally activated through T-cell regulatory elements downstream of BCL11B as a result of the t(5;14)(q35;q32). *Blood*. 2006;108(13):4198-4201. Prepublished on 2006/08/24 as DOI 10.1182/blood-2006-07-032953.

[34] Grossmann V, Bacher U, Kohlmann A, et al. EZH2 mutations and their association with PICALM-MLLT10 positive acute leukaemia. *Br J Haematol*. 2012;157(3):387-390. Prepublished on 2012/01/13 as DOI 10.1111/j.1365-2141.2011.08986.x.

[35] Okada Y, Jiang Q, Lemieux M, Jeannotte L, Su L, Zhang Y. Leukaemic transformation by CALM-AF10 involves upregulation of Hoxa5 by hDOT1L. *Nat Cell Biol*. 2006;8(9): 1017-1024. Prepublished on 2006/08/22 as DOI 10.1038/ncb1464.

[36] Hagemeijer A, Graux C. ABL1 rearrangements in T-cell acute lymphoblastic leukemia. *Genes Chromosomes Cancer*. 2010;49(4):299-308. Prepublished on 2010/01/15 as DOI 10.1002/gcc.20743.

[37] Zipfel PA, Zhang W, Quiroz M, Pendergast AM. Requirement for Abl kinases in T cell receptor signaling. *Curr Biol*. 2004;14(14):1222-1231. Prepublished on 2004/07/23 as DOI 10.1016/j.cub.2004.07.021.

[38] Flex E, Petrangeli V, Stella L, et al. Somatically acquired JAK1 mutations in adult acute lymphoblastic leukemia. *J Exp Med*. 2008;205(4):751-758. Prepublished on 2008/03/26 as DOI 10.1084/jem.20072182.

[39] Otsubo K, Kanegane H, Eguchi M, et al. ETV6-ARNT fusion in a patient with childhood T lymphoblastic leukemia. *Cancer Genet Cytogenet*. 2010;202(1):22-26. Prepublished on 2010/09/02 as DOI 10.1016/j.cancergencyto.2010.07.121.

[40] Fizzotti M, Cimino G, Pisegna S, et al. Detection of homozygous deletions of the cyclin-dependent kinase 4 inhibitor (p16) gene in acute lymphoblastic leukemia and association with adverse prognostic features. *Blood*. 1995;85(10):2685-2690. Prepublished on 1995/05/15 as DOI.

[41] Sulong S, Moorman AV, Irving JA, et al. A comprehensive analysis of the CDKN2A gene in childhood acute lymphoblastic leukemia reveals genomic deletion, copy

number neutral loss of heterozygosity, and association with specific cytogenetic subgroups. *Blood*. 2009;113(1):100-107. Prepublished on 2008/10/08 as DOI 10.1182/blood-2008-07-166801.

[42] Yamada Y, Hatta Y, Murata K, et al. Deletions of p15 and/or p16 genes as a poor-prognosis factor in adult T-cell leukemia. *J Clin Oncol*. 1997;15(5):1778-1785. Prepublished on 1997/05/01 as DOI.

[43] Daser A, Rabbitts TH. Extending the repertoire of the mixed-lineage leukemia gene MLL in leukemogenesis. *Genes Dev*. 2004;18(9):965-974. Prepublished on 2004/05/11 as DOI 10.1101/gad.1195504.

[44] Turkmen S, Timmermann B, Bartels G, et al. Involvement of the MLL gene in adult T-lymphoblastic leukemia. *Genes Chromosomes Cancer*. 2012. Prepublished on 2012/08/29 as DOI 10.1002/gcc.21996.

[45] O'Neil J, Calvo J, McKenna K, et al. Activating Notch1 mutations in mouse models of T-ALL. *Blood*. 2006;107(2):781-785. Prepublished on 2005/09/17 as DOI 10.1182/blood-2005-06-2553.

[46] Weng AP, Ferrando AA, Lee W, et al. Activating mutations of NOTCH1 in human T cell acute lymphoblastic leukemia. *Science*. 2004;306(5694):269-271. Prepublished on 2004/10/09 as DOI 10.1126/science.1102160.

[47] Asnafi V, Buzyn A, Le Noir S, et al. NOTCH1/FBXW7 mutation identifies a large subgroup with favorable outcome in adult T-cell acute lymphoblastic leukemia (T-ALL): a Group for Research on Adult Acute Lymphoblastic Leukemia (GRAALL) study. *Blood*. 2009;113(17):3918-3924. Prepublished on 2008/12/26 as DOI 10.1182/blood-2008-10-184069.

[48] Breit S, Stanulla M, Flohr T, et al. Activating NOTCH1 mutations predict favorable early treatment response and long-term outcome in childhood precursor T-cell lymphoblastic leukemia. *Blood*. 2006;108(4):1151-1157. Prepublished on 2006/04/15 as DOI 10.1182/blood-2005-12-4956.

[49] Larson Gedman A, Chen Q, Kugel Desmoulin S, et al. The impact of NOTCH1, FBW7 and PTEN mutations on prognosis and downstream signaling in pediatric T-cell acute lymphoblastic leukemia: a report from the Children's Oncology Group. *Leukemia*. 2009;23(8):1417-1425. Prepublished on 2009/04/03 as DOI 10.1038/leu.2009.64.

[50] Artavanis-Tsakonas S. The molecular biology of the Notch locus and the fine tuning of differentiation in Drosophila. *Trends Genet*. 1988;4(4):95-100. Prepublished on 1988/04/01 as DOI.

[51] Sambandam A, Maillard I, Zediak VP, et al. Notch signaling controls the generation and differentiation of early T lineage progenitors. *Nat Immunol*. 2005;6(7):663-670. Prepublished on 2005/06/14 as DOI 10.1038/ni1216.

[52] Ellisen LW, Bird J, West DC, et al. TAN-1, the human homolog of the Drosophila notch gene, is broken by chromosomal translocations in T lymphoblastic neoplasms. *Cell.* 1991;66(4):649-661. Prepublished on 1991/08/23 as DOI.

[53] Bellavia D, Checquolo S, Campese AF, Felli MP, Gulino A, Screpanti I. Notch3: from subtle structural differences to functional diversity. *Oncogene.* 2008;27(38):5092-5098. Prepublished on 2008/09/02 as DOI 10.1038/onc.2008.230.

[54] Rohn JL, Lauring AS, Linenberger ML, Overbaugh J. Transduction of Notch2 in feline leukemia virus-induced thymic lymphoma. *J Virol.* 1996;70(11):8071-8080. Prepublished on 1996/11/01 as DOI.

[55] Artavanis-Tsakonas S, Rand MD, Lake RJ. Notch signaling: cell fate control and signal integration in development. *Science.* 1999;284(5415):770-776. Prepublished on 1999/04/30 as DOI.

[56] Gupta-Rossi N, Le Bail O, Gonen H, et al. Functional interaction between SEL-10, an F-box protein, and the nuclear form of activated Notch1 receptor. *J Biol Chem.* 2001;276(37):34371-34378. Prepublished on 2001/06/27 as DOI 10.1074/jbc.M101343200.

[57] Hubbard EJ, Wu G, Kitajewski J, Greenwald I. sel-10, a negative regulator of lin-12 activity in Caenorhabditis elegans, encodes a member of the CDC4 family of proteins. *Genes Dev.* 1997;11(23):3182-3193. Prepublished on 1998/02/12 as DOI.

[58] Maser RS, Choudhury B, Campbell PJ, et al. Chromosomally unstable mouse tumours have genomic alterations similar to diverse human cancers. *Nature.* 2007;447(7147): 966-971. Prepublished on 2007/05/23 as DOI 10.1038/nature05886.

[59] O'Neil J, Grim J, Strack P, et al. FBW7 mutations in leukemic cells mediate NOTCH pathway activation and resistance to gamma-secretase inhibitors. *J Exp Med.* 2007;204(8):1813-1824. Prepublished on 2007/07/25 as DOI 10.1084/jem.20070876.

[60] Tetzlaff MT, Yu W, Li M, et al. Defective cardiovascular development and elevated cyclin E and Notch proteins in mice lacking the Fbw7 F-box protein. *Proc Natl Acad Sci U S A.* 2004;101(10):3338-3345. Prepublished on 2004/02/10 as DOI 10.1073/pnas. 0307875101.

[61] Thompson BJ, Buonamici S, Sulis ML, et al. The SCFFBW7 ubiquitin ligase complex as a tumor suppressor in T cell leukemia. *J Exp Med.* 2007;204(8):1825-1835. Prepublished on 2007/07/25 as DOI 10.1084/jem.20070872.

[62] Guruharsha KG, Kankel MW, Artavanis-Tsakonas S. The Notch signalling system: recent insights into the complexity of a conserved pathway. *Nat Rev Genet.* 2012;13(9): 654-666. Prepublished on 2012/08/08 as DOI 10.1038/nrg3272.

[63] Barrick D, Kopan R. The Notch transcription activation complex makes its move. *Cell.* 2006;124(5):883-885. Prepublished on 2006/03/15 as DOI 10.1016/j.cell.2006.02.028.

[64] Palomero T, Lim WK, Odom DT, et al. NOTCH1 directly regulates c-MYC and activates a feed-forward-loop transcriptional network promoting leukemic cell growth. *Proc Natl*

Acad Sci U S A. 2006;103(48):18261-18266. Prepublished on 2006/11/23 as DOI 10.1073/pnas.0606108103.

[65]   Klinakis A, Szabolcs M, Politi K, Kiaris H, Artavanis-Tsakonas S, Efstratiadis A. Myc is a Notch1 transcriptional target and a requisite for Notch1-induced mammary tumorigenesis in mice. *Proc Natl Acad Sci U S A*. 2006;103(24):9262-9267. Prepublished on 2006/06/06 as DOI 10.1073/pnas.0603371103.

[66]   Sharma VM, Calvo JA, Draheim KM, et al. Notch1 contributes to mouse T-cell leukemia by directly inducing the expression of c-myc. *Mol Cell Biol*. 2006;26(21):8022-8031. Prepublished on 2006/09/07 as DOI 10.1128/MCB.01091-06.

[67]   Weng AP, Millholland JM, Yashiro-Ohtani Y, et al. c-Myc is an important direct target of Notch1 in T-cell acute lymphoblastic leukemia/lymphoma. *Genes Dev*. 2006;20(15): 2096-2109. Prepublished on 2006/07/19 as DOI 10.1101/gad.1450406.

[68]   Vilimas T, Mascarenhas J, Palomero T, et al. Targeting the NF-kappaB signaling pathway in Notch1-induced T-cell leukemia. *Nat Med*. 2007;13(1):70-77. Prepublished on 2006/12/19 as DOI 10.1038/nm1524.

[69]   Palomero T, Sulis ML, Cortina M, et al. Mutational loss of PTEN induces resistance to NOTCH1 inhibition in T-cell leukemia. *Nat Med*. 2007;13(10):1203-1210. Prepublished on 2007/09/18 as DOI 10.1038/nm1636.

[70]   Medyouf H, Alcalde H, Berthier C, et al. Targeting calcineurin activation as a thera- peutic strategy for T-cell acute lymphoblastic leukemia. *Nat Med*. 2007;13(6):736-741. Prepublished on 2007/05/23 as DOI 10.1038/nm1588.

[71]   Kox C, Zimmermann M, Stanulla M, et al. The favorable effect of activating NOTCH1 receptor mutations on long-term outcome in T-ALL patients treated on the ALL-BFM 2000 protocol can be separated from FBXW7 loss of function. *Leukemia*. 2010;24(12): 2005-2013. Prepublished on 2010/10/15 as DOI 10.1038/leu.2010.203.

[72]   Gutierrez A, Sanda T, Grebliunaite R, et al. High frequency of PTEN, PI3K, and AKT abnormalities in T-cell acute lymphoblastic leukemia. *Blood*. 2009;114(3):647-650. Prepublished on 2009/05/22 as DOI 10.1182/blood-2009-02-206722.

[73]   Drexler HG. Review of alterations of the cyclin-dependent kinase inhibitor INK4 family genes p15, p16, p18 and p19 in human leukemia-lymphoma cells. *Leukemia*. 1998;12(6): 845-859. Prepublished on 1998/06/25 as DOI.

[74]   Ruas M, Peters G. The p16INK4a/CDKN2A tumor suppressor and its relatives. *Biochim Biophys Acta*. 1998;1378(2):F115-177. Prepublished on 1998/11/21 as DOI.

[75]   Remke M, Pfister S, Kox C, et al. High-resolution genomic profiling of childhood T- ALL reveals frequent copy-number alterations affecting the TGF-beta and PI3K-AKT pathways and deletions at 6q15-16.1 as a genomic marker for unfavorable early treatment response. *Blood*. 2009;114(5):1053-1062. Prepublished on 2009/05/02 as DOI 10.1182/blood-2008-10-186536.

[76] Van Vlierberghe P, Palomero T, Khiabanian H, et al. PHF6 mutations in T-cell acute lymphoblastic leukemia. *Nat Genet.* 2010;42(4):338-342. Prepublished on 2010/03/17 as DOI 10.1038/ng.542.

[77] Todd MA, Picketts DJ. PHF6 Interacts with the Nucleosome Remodeling and Deacetylation (NuRD) Complex. *J Proteome Res.* 2012;11(8):4326-4337. Prepublished on 2012/06/23 as DOI 10.1021/pr3004369.

[78] Renneville A, Kaltenbach S, Clappier E, et al. Wilms tumor 1 (WT1) gene mutations in pediatric T-cell malignancies. *Leukemia.* 2010;24(2):476-480. Prepublished on 2009/10/23 as DOI 10.1038/leu.2009.221.

[79] Tosello V, Mansour MR, Barnes K, et al. WT1 mutations in T-ALL. *Blood.* 2009;114(5):1038-1045. Prepublished on 2009/06/06 as DOI 10.1182/blood-2008-12-192039.

[80] Dame C, Kirschner KM, Bartz KV, Wallach T, Hussels CS, Scholz H. Wilms tumor suppressor, Wt1, is a transcriptional activator of the erythropoietin gene. *Blood.* 2006;107(11):4282-4290. Prepublished on 2006/02/10 as DOI 10.1182/blood-2005-07-2889.

[81] Gutierrez A, Sanda T, Ma W, et al. Inactivation of LEF1 in T-cell acute lymphoblastic leukemia. *Blood.* 2010;115(14):2845-2851. Prepublished on 2010/02/04 as DOI 10.1182/blood-2009-07-234377.

[82] Schindler C, Levy DE, Decker T. JAK-STAT signaling: from interferons to cytokines. *J Biol Chem.* 2007;282(28):20059-20063. Prepublished on 2007/05/16 as DOI 10.1074/jbc.R700016200.

[83] Yamaoka K, Saharinen P, Pesu M, Holt VE, 3rd, Silvennoinen O, O'Shea JJ. The Janus kinases (Jaks). *Genome Biol.* 2004;5(12):253. Prepublished on 2004/12/04 as DOI 10.1186/gb-2004-5-12-253.

[84] Kleppe M, Tousseyn T, Geissinger E, et al. Mutation analysis of the tyrosine phosphatase PTPN2 in Hodgkin's lymphoma and T-cell non-Hodgkin's lymphoma. *Haematologica.* 2011;96(11):1723-1727. Prepublished on 2011/07/28 as DOI 10.3324/haematol.2011.041921.

[85] Zenatti PP, Ribeiro D, Li W, et al. Oncogenic IL7R gain-of-function mutations in childhood T-cell acute lymphoblastic leukemia. *Nat Genet.* 2011;43(10):932-939. Prepublished on 2011/09/06 as DOI 10.1038/ng.924.

[86] Fry TJ, Mackall CL. The many faces of IL-7: from lymphopoiesis to peripheral T cell maintenance. *J Immunol.* 2005;174(11):6571-6576. Prepublished on 2005/05/21 as DOI.

[87] Jiang Q, Li WQ, Aiello FB, et al. Cell biology of IL-7, a key lymphotrophin. *Cytokine Growth Factor Rev.* 2005;16(4-5):513-533. Prepublished on 2005/07/06 as DOI 10.1016/j.cytogfr.2005.05.004.

[88] Peschon JJ, Morrissey PJ, Grabstein KH, et al. Early lymphocyte expansion is severely impaired in interleukin 7 receptor-deficient mice. *J Exp Med*. 1994;180(5):1955-1960. Prepublished on 1994/11/01 as DOI.

[89] von Freeden-Jeffry U, Vieira P, Lucian LA, McNeil T, Burdach SE, Murray R. Lymphopenia in interleukin (IL)-7 gene-deleted mice identifies IL-7 as a nonredundant cytokine. *J Exp Med*. 1995;181(4):1519-1526. Prepublished on 1995/04/01 as DOI.

[90] Puel A, Ziegler SF, Buckley RH, Leonard WJ. Defective IL7R expression in T(-)B(+)NK(+) severe combined immunodeficiency. *Nat Genet*. 1998;20(4):394-397. Prepublished on 1998/12/08 as DOI 10.1038/3877.

[91] Gonzalez-Garcia S, Garcia-Peydro M, Martin-Gayo E, et al. CSL-MAML-dependent Notch1 signaling controls T lineage-specific IL-7R{alpha} gene expression in early human thymopoiesis and leukemia. *J Exp Med*. 2009;206(4):779-791. Prepublished on 2009/04/08 as DOI 10.1084/jem.20081922.

[92] Kleppe M, Lahortiga I, El Chaar T, et al. Deletion of the protein tyrosine phosphatase gene PTPN2 in T-cell acute lymphoblastic leukemia. *Nat Genet*. 2010;42(6):530-535. Prepublished on 2010/05/18 as DOI 10.1038/ng.587.

[93] Abu-Duhier FM, Goodeve AC, Wilson GA, Care RS, Peake IR, Reilly JT. Identification of novel FLT-3 Asp835 mutations in adult acute myeloid leukaemia. *Br J Haematol*. 2001;113(4):983-988. Prepublished on 2001/07/10 as DOI.

[94] Nakao M, Yokota S, Iwai T, et al. Internal tandem duplication of the flt3 gene found in acute myeloid leukemia. *Leukemia*. 1996;10(12):1911-1918. Prepublished on 1996/12/01 as DOI.

[95] Yamamoto Y, Kiyoi H, Nakano Y, et al. Activating mutation of D835 within the activation loop of FLT3 in human hematologic malignancies. *Blood*. 2001;97(8): 2434-2439. Prepublished on 2001/04/06 as DOI.

[96] Mansur MB, Emerenciano M, Splendore A, Brewer L, Hassan R, Pombo-de-Oliveira MS. T-cell lymphoblastic leukemia in early childhood presents NOTCH1 mutations and MLL rearrangements. *Leuk Res*. 2010;34(4):483-486. Prepublished on 2009/07/28 as DOI 10.1016/j.leukres.2009.06.026.

[97] Nakao M, Janssen JW, Erz D, Seriu T, Bartram CR. Tandem duplication of the FLT3 gene in acute lymphoblastic leukemia: a marker for the monitoring of minimal residual disease. *Leukemia*. 2000;14(3):522-524. Prepublished on 2000/03/17 as DOI.

[98] Van Vlierberghe P, Meijerink JP, Stam RW, et al. Activating FLT3 mutations in CD4+/CD8- pediatric T-cell acute lymphoblastic leukemias. *Blood*. 2005;106(13):4414-4415. Prepublished on 2005/12/06 as DOI 10.1182/blood-2005-06-2267.

[99] Paietta E, Ferrando AA, Neuberg D, et al. Activating FLT3 mutations in CD117/KIT(+) T-cell acute lymphoblastic leukemias. *Blood*. 2004;104(2):558-560. Prepublished on 2004/03/27 as DOI 10.1182/blood-2004-01-0168.

[100] Williams AB, Nguyen B, Li L, et al. Mutations of FLT3/ITD confer resistance to multiple tyrosine kinase inhibitors. *Leukemia*. 2012. Prepublished on 2012/08/04 as DOI 10.1038/leu.2012.191.

[101] Gutierrez A, Kentsis A, Sanda T, et al. The BCL11B tumor suppressor is mutated across the major molecular subtypes of T-cell acute lymphoblastic leukemia. *Blood*. 2011;118(15):4169-4173. Prepublished on 2011/09/01 as DOI 10.1182/blood-2010-11-318873.

[102] Dik WA, Pike-Overzet K, Weerkamp F, et al. New insights on human T cell development by quantitative T cell receptor gene rearrangement studies and gene expression profiling. *J Exp Med*. 2005;201(11):1715-1723. Prepublished on 2005/06/02 as DOI 10.1084/jem.20042524.

[103] Huang X, Shen Q, Chen S, et al. Gene expression profiles in BCL11B-siRNA treated malignant T cells. *J Hematol Oncol*. 2011;4:23. Prepublished on 2011/05/18 as DOI 10.1186/1756-8722-4-23.

[104] Kastner P, Chan S, Vogel WK, et al. Bcl11b represses a mature T-cell gene expression program in immature CD4(+)CD8(+) thymocytes. *Eur J Immunol*. 2010;40(8):2143-2154. Prepublished on 2010/06/15 as DOI 10.1002/eji.200940258.

[105] Przybylski GK, Dik WA, Wanzeck J, et al. Disruption of the BCL11B gene through inv(14)(q11.2q32.31) results in the expression of BCL11B-TRDC fusion transcripts and is associated with the absence of wild-type BCL11B transcripts in T-ALL. *Leukemia*. 2005;19(2):201-208. Prepublished on 2005/01/26 as DOI 10.1038/sj.leu.2403619.

[106] Robbins SH, Walzer T, Dembele D, et al. Novel insights into the relationships between dendritic cell subsets in human and mouse revealed by genome-wide expression profiling. *Genome Biol*. 2008;9(1):R17. Prepublished on 2008/01/26 as DOI 10.1186/gb-2008-9-1-r17.

[107] Yokota S, Nakao M, Horiike S, et al. Mutational analysis of the N-ras gene in acute lymphoblastic leukemia: a study of 125 Japanese pediatric cases. *Int J Hematol*. 1998;67(4):379-387. Prepublished on 1998/08/08 as DOI.

[108] Ferrando AA, Neuberg DS, Staunton J, et al. Gene expression signatures define novel oncogenic pathways in T cell acute lymphoblastic leukemia. *Cancer Cell*. 2002;1(1):75-87. Prepublished on 2002/06/28 as DOI.

[109] Coustan-Smith E, Mullighan CG, Onciu M, et al. Early T-cell precursor leukaemia: a subtype of very high-risk acute lymphoblastic leukaemia. *Lancet Oncol*. 2009;10(2):147-156. Prepublished on 2009/01/17 as DOI 10.1016/S1470-2045(08)70314-0.

[110] Mavrakis KJ, Van Der Meulen J, Wolfe AL, et al. A cooperative microRNA-tumor suppressor gene network in acute T-cell lymphoblastic leukemia (T-ALL). *Nat Genet*. 2011;43(7):673-678. Prepublished on 2011/06/07 as DOI 10.1038/ng.858.

[111] Begley CG, Aplan PD, Denning SM, Haynes BF, Waldmann TA, Kirsch IR. The gene SCL is expressed during early hematopoiesis and encodes a differentiation-related

DNA-binding motif. *Proc Natl Acad Sci U S A*. 1989;86(24):10128-10132. Prepublished on 1989/12/01 as DOI.

[112] Bash RO, Hall S, Timmons CF, et al. Does activation of the TAL1 gene occur in a majority of patients with T-cell acute lymphoblastic leukemia? A pediatric oncology group study. *Blood*. 1995;86(2):666-676. Prepublished on 1995/07/15 as DOI.

[113] Cantor AB, Orkin SH. Transcriptional regulation of erythropoiesis: an affair involving multiple partners. *Oncogene*. 2002;21(21):3368-3376. Prepublished on 2002/05/29 as DOI 10.1038/sj.onc.1205326.

[114] Hsu HL, Wadman I, Baer R. Formation of in vivo complexes between the TAL1 and E2A polypeptides of leukemic T cells. *Proc Natl Acad Sci U S A*. 1994;91(8):3181-3185. Prepublished on 1994/04/12 as DOI.

[115] Anantharaman A, Lin IJ, Barrow J, et al. Role of helix-loop-helix proteins during differentiation of erythroid cells. *Mol Cell Biol*. 2011;31(7):1332-1343. Prepublished on 2011/02/02 as DOI 10.1128/MCB.01186-10.

[116] El Omari K, Hoosdally SJ, Tuladhar K, et al. Structure of the leukemia oncogene LMO2: implications for the assembly of a hematopoietic transcription factor complex. *Blood*. 2011;117(7):2146-2156. Prepublished on 2010/11/16 as DOI 10.1182/blood-2010-07-293357.

[117] Lecuyer E, Hoang T. SCL: from the origin of hematopoiesis to stem cells and leukemia. *Exp Hematol*. 2004;32(1):11-24. Prepublished on 2004/01/17 as DOI.

[118] Sanda T, Lawton LN, Barrasa MI, et al. Core Transcriptional Regulatory Circuit Controlled by the TAL1 Complex in Human T Cell Acute Lymphoblastic Leukemia. *Cancer Cell*. 2012;22(2):209-221. Prepublished on 2012/08/18 as DOI 10.1016/j.ccr.2012.06.007.

[119] Hsu HL, Cheng JT, Chen Q, Baer R. Enhancer-binding activity of the tal-1 oncoprotein in association with the E47/E12 helix-loop-helix proteins. *Mol Cell Biol*. 1991;11(6):3037-3042. Prepublished on 1991/06/01 as DOI.

[120] Park ST, Sun XH. The Tal1 oncoprotein inhibits E47-mediated transcription. Mechanism of inhibition. *J Biol Chem*. 1998;273(12):7030-7037. Prepublished on 1998/04/18 as DOI.

[121] Voronova AF, Lee F. The E2A and tal-1 helix-loop-helix proteins associate in vivo and are modulated by Id proteins during interleukin 6-induced myeloid differentiation. *Proc Natl Acad Sci U S A*. 1994;91(13):5952-5956. Prepublished on 1994/06/21 as DOI.

[122] Kassouf MT, Hughes JR, Taylor S, et al. Genome-wide identification of TAL1's functional targets: insights into its mechanisms of action in primary erythroid cells. *Genome Res*. 2010;20(8):1064-1083. Prepublished on 2010/06/23 as DOI 10.1101/gr.104935.110.

[123] Hu X, Li X, Valverde K, et al. LSD1-mediated epigenetic modification is required for TAL1 function and hematopoiesis. *Proc Natl Acad Sci U S A.* 2009;106(25):10141-10146. Prepublished on 2009/06/06 as DOI 10.1073/pnas.0900437106.

[124] Palomero T, Odom DT, O'Neil J, et al. Transcriptional regulatory networks downstream of TAL1/SCL in T-cell acute lymphoblastic leukemia. *Blood.* 2006;108(3):986-992. Prepublished on 2006/04/20 as DOI 10.1182/blood-2005-08-3482.

[125] Kusy S, Gerby B, Goardon N, et al. NKX3.1 is a direct TAL1 target gene that mediates proliferation of TAL1-expressing human T cell acute lymphoblastic leukemia. *J Exp Med.* 2010;207(10):2141-2156. Prepublished on 2010/09/22 as DOI 10.1084/jem.20100745.

[126] Ono Y, Fukuhara N, Yoshie O. TAL1 and LIM-only proteins synergistically induce retinaldehyde dehydrogenase 2 expression in T-cell acute lymphoblastic leukemia by acting as cofactors for GATA3. *Mol Cell Biol.* 1998;18(12):6939-6950. Prepublished on 1998/11/20 as DOI.

[127] Huang S, Qiu Y, Shi Y, Xu Z, Brandt SJ. P/CAF-mediated acetylation regulates the function of the basic helix-loop-helix transcription factor TAL1/SCL. *EMBO J.* 2000;19(24):6792-6803. Prepublished on 2000/12/16 as DOI 10.1093/emboj/19.24.6792.

[128] Huang S, Qiu Y, Stein RW, Brandt SJ. p300 functions as a transcriptional coactivator for the TAL1/SCL oncoprotein. *Oncogene.* 1999;18(35):4958-4967. Prepublished on 1999/09/22 as DOI 10.1038/sj.onc.1202889.

[129] Giroux S, Kaushik AL, Capron C, et al. lyl-1 and tal-1/scl, two genes encoding closely related bHLH transcription factors, display highly overlapping expression patterns during cardiovascular and hematopoietic ontogeny. *Gene Expr Patterns.* 2007;7(3): 215-226. Prepublished on 2006/11/23 as DOI 10.1016/j.modgep.2006.10.004.

[130] Boehm T, Baer R, Lavenir I, et al. The mechanism of chromosomal translocation t(11;14) involving the T-cell receptor C delta locus on human chromosome 14q11 and a transcribed region of chromosome 11p15. *EMBO J.* 1988;7(2):385-394. Prepublished on 1988/02/01 as DOI.

[131] Boehm T, Foroni L, Kaneko Y, Perutz MF, Rabbitts TH. The rhombotin family of cysteine-rich LIM-domain oncogenes: distinct members are involved in T-cell translocations to human chromosomes 11p15 and 11p13. *Proc Natl Acad Sci U S A.* 1991;88(10): 4367-4371. Prepublished on 1991/05/15 as DOI.

[132] Royer-Pokora B, Loos U, Ludwig WD. TTG-2, a new gene encoding a cysteine-rich protein with the LIM motif, is overexpressed in acute T-cell leukaemia with the t(11;14) (p13;q11). *Oncogene.* 1991;6(10):1887-1893. Prepublished on 1991/10/01 as DOI.

[133] Osada H, Grutz G, Axelson H, Forster A, Rabbitts TH. Association of erythroid transcription factors: complexes involving the LIM protein RBTN2 and the zinc-finger protein GATA1. *Proc Natl Acad Sci U S A.* 1995;92(21):9585-9589. Prepublished on 1995/10/10 as DOI.

[134] Valge-Archer V, Forster A, Rabbitts TH. The LMO1 and LDB1 proteins interact in human T cell acute leukaemia with the chromosomal translocation t(11;14)(p15;q11). *Oncogene*. 1998;17(24):3199-3202. Prepublished on 1999/01/01 as DOI 10.1038/sj.onc. 1202353.

[135] Valge-Archer VE, Osada H, Warren AJ, et al. The LIM protein RBTN2 and the basic helix-loop-helix protein TAL1 are present in a complex in erythroid cells. *Proc Natl Acad Sci U S A*. 1994;91(18):8617-8621. Prepublished on 1994/08/30 as DOI.

[136] Wadman IA, Osada H, Grutz GG, et al. The LIM-only protein Lmo2 is a bridging molecule assembling an erythroid, DNA-binding complex which includes the TAL1, E47, GATA-1 and Ldb1/NLI proteins. *EMBO J*. 1997;16(11):3145-3157. Prepublished on 1997/06/02 as DOI 10.1093/emboj/16.11.3145.

[137] Grutz GG, Bucher K, Lavenir I, Larson T, Larson R, Rabbitts TH. The oncogenic T cell LIM-protein Lmo2 forms part of a DNA-binding complex specifically in immature T cells. *EMBO J*. 1998;17(16):4594-4605. Prepublished on 1998/08/26 as DOI 10.1093/emboj/17.16.4594.

[138] Chervinsky DS, Zhao XF, Lam DH, Ellsworth M, Gross KW, Aplan PD. Disordered T-cell development and T-cell malignancies in SCL LMO1 double-transgenic mice: parallels with E2A-deficient mice. *Mol Cell Biol*. 1999;19(7):5025-5035. Prepublished on 1999/06/22 as DOI.

[139] Larson RC, Lavenir I, Larson TA, et al. Protein dimerization between Lmo2 (Rbtn2) and Tal1 alters thymocyte development and potentiates T cell tumorigenesis in transgenic mice. *EMBO J*. 1996;15(5):1021-1027. Prepublished on 1996/03/01 as DOI.

[140] Tremblay M, Tremblay CS, Herblot S, et al. Modeling T-cell acute lymphoblastic leukemia induced by the SCL and LMO1 oncogenes. *Genes Dev*. 2010;24(11):1093-1105. Prepublished on 2010/06/03 as DOI 10.1101/gad.1897910.

[141] Argiropoulos B, Humphries RK. Hox genes in hematopoiesis and leukemogenesis. *Oncogene*. 2007;26(47):6766-6776. Prepublished on 2007/10/16 as DOI 10.1038/sj.onc. 1210760.

[142] Gehring WJ, Qian YQ, Billeter M, et al. Homeodomain-DNA recognition. *Cell*. 1994;78(2):211-223. Prepublished on 1994/07/29 as DOI.

[143] Owens BM, Hawley RG. HOX and non-HOX homeobox genes in leukemic hemato-poiesis. *Stem Cells*. 2002;20(5):364-379. Prepublished on 2002/09/28 as DOI 10.1634/stemcells.20-5-364.

[144] Su X, Drabkin H, Clappier E, et al. Transforming potential of the T-cell acute lympho-blastic leukemia-associated homeobox genes HOXA13, TLX1, and TLX3. *Genes Chromosomes Cancer*. 2006;45(9):846-855. Prepublished on 2006/06/29 as DOI 10.1002/gcc.20348.

[145] Roberts CW, Shutter JR, Korsmeyer SJ. Hox11 controls the genesis of the spleen. *Nature*. 1994;368(6473):747-749. Prepublished on 1994/04/21 as DOI 10.1038/368747a0.

[146] Dixon DN, Izon DJ, Dagger S, et al. TLX1/HOX11 transcription factor inhibits differentiation and promotes a non-haemopoietic phenotype in murine bone marrow cells. *Br J Haematol.* 2007;138(1):54-67. Prepublished on 2007/06/09 as DOI 10.1111/j.1365-2141.2007.06626.x.

[147] Hawley RG, Fong AZ, Lu M, Hawley TS. The HOX11 homeobox-containing gene of human leukemia immortalizes murine hematopoietic precursors. *Oncogene.* 1994;9(1):1-12. Prepublished on 1994/01/01 as DOI.

[148] Hawley RG, Fong AZ, Reis MD, Zhang N, Lu M, Hawley TS. Transforming function of the HOX11/TCL3 homeobox gene. *Cancer Res.* 1997;57(2):337-345. Prepublished on 1997/01/15 as DOI.

[149] Riz I, Hawley TS, Luu TV, Lee NH, Hawley RG. TLX1 and NOTCH coregulate transcription in T cell acute lymphoblastic leukemia cells. *Mol Cancer.* 2010;9:181. Prepublished on 2010/07/14 as DOI 10.1186/1476-4598-9-181.

[150] Ntziachristos P, Tsirigos A, Van Vlierberghe P, et al. Genetic inactivation of the polycomb repressive complex 2 in T cell acute lymphoblastic leukemia. *Nat Med.* 2012;18(2):298-301. Prepublished on 2012/01/13 as DOI 10.1038/nm.2651.

[151] Kraszewska MD, Dawidowska M, Larmonie NS, et al. DNA methylation pattern is altered in childhood T-cell acute lymphoblastic leukemia patients as compared with normal thymic subsets: insights into CpG island methylator phenotype in T-ALL. *Leukemia.* 2012;26(2):367-371. Prepublished on 2011/08/13 as DOI 10.1038/leu.2011.208.

[152] Pui CH, Mullighan CG, Evans WE, Relling MV. Pediatric acute lymphoblastic leukemia: where are we going and how do we get there? *Blood.* 2012;120(6):1165-1174. Prepublished on 2012/06/26 as DOI 10.1182/blood-2012-05-378943.

Chapter 2

T- and NK/T-Cell Leukemia in East Asia

Tsung-Hsien Lin, Yen-Chuan Hsieh,
Sheng-Tsung Chang and Shih-Sung Chuang

Additional information is available at the end of the chapter

1. Introduction

The relative frequency of lymphoma types varies in different geographic region. Human T-cell lymphotropic virus type I (HTLV-I) infection is endemic in south-western Japan which leads to a high frequency of adult T-cell leukemia/lymphoma (ATLL). As compared to the West, East Asian countries have higher relative frequencies of T- and natural killer (NK)-cell lymphomas, which account for about 15-20% of non-Hodgkin lymphoma after excluding ATLL in some Japanese series [1-5]. Accordingly, a higher frequency of T- and NK/T-cell leukemia would be expected in East Asia. As compared to B-cell lymphomas, T- and NK/T-cell neoplasms more frequently occur at extranodal locations, and may occasionally present as leukemia, either with or without concomitant lymphoma.

There are around 20 entities and variants of T- and NK/T-cell neoplasms in the 4th edition of World Health Organization (WHO) classification of lymphoid neoplasms [6]. Table 1 lists the T- and NK/T-cell neoplasms which may have leukemic presentation. The first category comprises entities that are predominantly leukemic including T-cell prolymphocytic leukemia (T-PLL), T-cell large granular lymphocytic leukemia (T-LGLL) and aggressive NK-cell leukemia (ANKL). The second category includes neoplasms that frequently present with concurrent lymphoma and leukemia such as T lymphoblastic leukemia/lymphoma (T-LBL), ATLL and Sézary syndrome. The third category includes T-cell lymphoma with secondary peripheral blood involvement such as unspecified peripheral T-cell lymphoma (PTCL-NOS) progressing to a leukemic phase and very rarely extranodal NK/T-cell lymphoma (ENKTL) with peripheral blood involvement, which might overlap with ANKL [7]. In the East Asian region other than Japan, ATLL is extremely rare and the discussion on this entity is covered in the other chapters. Sézary syndrome is extremely rare in this region as well. Accordingly we will not discuss these two entities in this chapter.

A. Predominantly leukemic
1. T-cell prolymphocytic leukemia (T-PLL)
2. T-cell large granular lymphocytic leukemia (T-LGLL)
3. Aggressive NK-cell leukemia (ANKL)
B. Concurrent lymphoma/leukemia
1. T lymphoblastic lymphoma/leukemia (T-LBL)
2. Adult T-cell lymphoma/leukemia (ATLL)
3. Sézary syndrome
C. Lymphoma with secondary peripheral blood involvement
1. Peripheral T-cell lymphoma with peripheral blood involvement
2. Extranodal NK/T-cell lymphoma with peripheral blood involvement

Table 1. T- and NK/T-cell neoplasms with leukemic presentation.

There are very few reports systemically reviewing the whole spectrum of T- and NK/T-cell neoplasms with leukemic presentation in the East Asia. In a prospective study of chronic lymphoproliferative disorders in Hong Kong in an 18-month period from January 1995 to June 1996, there were a total of 34 cases of chronic lymphoproliferative disorder, estimated at 0.54 case per million populations per year, as compared to 245 new cases of acute myeloid leukemia in the same study period [8]. Of these 34 cases, the majority were B-cell neoplasms with the remaining 3 (9%) cases being T-cell leukemias including one case each of T-PLL, Sézary syndrome and T-LGLL [8]. In our recent retrospective study of 718 consecutive patients with lymphoid neoplasms in a single institution in Taiwan, the frequency of T- and NK/T-cell neoplasms with leukemic presentation was 13.1% (18 of 137 patients) [9]. Our study showed that cases with concurrent lymphoma, higher absolute leukemic cell counts, and elevated lactate dehydrogenase level carried a poorer prognosis. The survival of patients with leukemic presentation was dichotomous, with a very poor prognosis for patients with T-LBL, T-PLL, ANKL, ATLL in acute phase, and PTCL-NOS; while those with T-LGLL and ATLL in chronic phase had a favorable outcome.

Table 2 summarizes the relative frequency of various T- and NK/T-cell leukemia in different countries in the East Asia [1,4,9]. As mentioned previously, T- and NK/T-cell neoplasms account for 15-20% of lymphomas in this region. The relative frequency of T-LBL among T-cell neoplasms is low in Taiwan and Japan at less than 10%, but it is high at 23.77% (208 of 875 cases) in Korea, which is partly due to the inclusion of all lymphoid neoplasms including T-cell acute lymphoblastic leukemia in that Korean study [4]. T-PLL is very rare in all 3 countries with a relative frequency of less than 1% among T-cell neoplasms. T-LGLL and ANKL are also rare with a frequency of less than 1% except for a higher frequency of the former in Taiwan and the latter in Korea, respectively. The higher relative frequency of T-LGLL in our series in Taiwan is probably due to a higher interest of this entity in our laboratory with confirmation of suspicious cases by T-cell receptor (TCR) gene rearrangement and/or flow cytometry immunophenotyping (aberrancy in T-cell antigen expression or clonal by flow cytometric TCR-Vβ repertoire analysis) [10]. While in other pathology laboratories, such cases might either be unrecognized or diagnosed solely by hematologists without marrow trephine biopsy and thus not being enrolled in the pathology files for lymphoma analysis. In the following sections, we will discuss each specific T- and NK/T-cell neoplasm.

	Taiwan [9]	Japan-1A [1]	Japan-1B [1]	Japan-2 [5]	Korea [4]
T-cell/total neoplasms (%)	137/718 (19.08%)	796/3,194 (24.92%)	558/2,956 (18.88%)	287/1,552 (18.49%)	875/5,318 (16.45%)
T-LBL	2.92% (n=4)	6.91% (n=55)	9.86% (n=55)	6.62% (n=19)	23.77% (n=208)
T-PLL	0.73% (n=1)	0.25% (n=2)	0.36% (n=2)	0.35% (n=1)	0.57% (n=5)
T-LGL leukemia	5.10% (n=7)	0.25% (n=2)	0.36% (n=2)	-	0.23% (n=2)
ANKL	0.73% (n=1)	0.38% (n=3)	0.54% (n=3)	0.70% (n=2)	3.31% (n=29)
ATLL	2.92% (n=4)	29.90% (n=238)	Excluded	14.29% (n=41)	0.11% (n=1)

*Data of various T- and NK-cell neoplasms are presented as percentage (case number) among the total number of T- and NK-cell neoplasms in each country.

Columns Japan-1A and -1B are from the same reference with exclusion of ATLL cases in the column of Japan-1B.

Table 2. Relative frequency of various T- and NK/T-cell leukemia among T-cell neoplasms in representative East Asian countries.

2. T Lymphoblastic Leukemia/Lymphoma (T-LBL)

T-LBL is a rare neoplasm occurring more commonly in adolescents, accounting for 1-4% among malignant lymphomas in East Asia [1,2,4,5,9]. Patients with T-LBL usually present with a very high leukemic cell count (frequently over 150,000/µL), and often with a large mediastinal mass [9]. The diagnosis is often straightforward with typical clinical features and numerous blasts in the peripheral blood with a fine chromatin pattern and irregular nuclear contours (Fig. 1A). Phenotypically, the neoplastic cells express cytoplasmic but not surface CD3; and they frequently co-express CD4 and CD8. The most important and reliable immature cell marker is terminal deoxynucleotidyl transferase (TdT), which could be used either in immunohistochemistry or flow cytometry [11]. The other immature markers are CD1a, CD34 and CD99 [12,13]. Immunohistochemically, occasional cases of T-LBL may not express TdT, but instead, express CD34 and/or CD99 [14]. The immunophenotype of T-LBL and T-cell acute lymphoblastic leukemia are identical but differ in frequency, with a higher rate of later phases of development (cortical or mature immunophenotype) in T-LBL, which is probably reflecting the higher rate (> 90%) of mediastinal tumors [15].

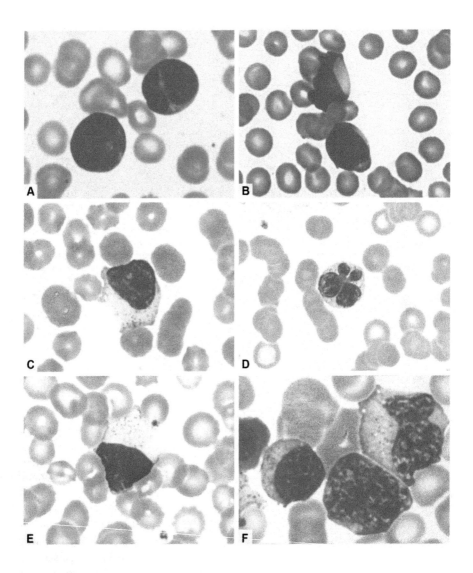

Figure 1. Photomicrographs of representative cases in the peripheral blood smear of A) T-LBL with indented nuclei, B) T-PLL of small cell variant without nucleoli, C) T-LGLL with usual LGL morphology containing azurophilic cytoplasmic granules, D) T-LGLL with atypical morphology characterized by irregular nuclear contours resembling a flower, E) reactive NK lymphocytosis and F), ANKL.

3. T-cell Prolymphocytic Leukemia (T-PLL)

T-PLL is rare, representing around 2% of mature lymphocytic leukemia in adults over the age of 30 in the West with a median age of 65 [16]. The main disease features are splenomegaly, lymphadenopathy, hepatomegaly, skin lesions, and a high leukocyte count comprising small to medium-sized nucleolated prolymphocytes with cytoplasmic protrusions or blebs but devoid of granules (Fig. 1B). Small cell variant with small, less typical cells and an indistinct nucleolus has been recognized in 20% cases [16]. T-PLLs account for less than 1% of T- and NK-cell lymphomas in East Asia. The clinical manifestations and immunophenotype of T-PLL in Japan are similar to those of the Western cases [17-19]. However, there is a significantly higher frequency of tumor cells in Japanese cases expressing HLA-DR than that of Western cases [17]. Chromosome 14q11 abnormality and trisomy 8q, which are frequently seen in T-PLL of Western countries (70-80%), are not common in Japan [18]. Furthermore, a substantial number of T-PLL cases in Japan shows abnormal expression of TCL1A, probably due to rearrangement of *TCL1* gene, which may serve as a useful marker for diagnosing T-PLL [19]. In contrast to the aggressive clinical courses observed in Western T-PLL patients, Kameoka et al. reported that 6 out of 13 Japanese patients experienced an indolent course. Interestingly, the clinical course closely correlated with morphology; 86% cases of typical morphology were aggressive, whereas 83% of small-cell variant were indolent [17]. Studies on more cases are needed to see if Japanese T-PLL constitutes a variant of T-PLL. In East Asia countries other than Japan, there are only scanty reports on T-PLL, either included in a small case series or as a single case report [9, 20].

4. T-cell Large Granular Lymphocytic Leukemia (T-LGLL)

Large granular lymphocytes (LGLs) are medium to large-sized lymphocytes with azurophilic cytoplasmic granules that normally comprise 10-15% of the peripheral blood mononuclear cells (PBMCs) and serve as the main effector cells of cell-mediated cytotoxicity. The majority (85%) of these LGLs are NK-cells with the remaining minority being CD8-positive cytotoxic T-cells [21]. LGL lymphoproliferation may be reactive or neoplastic; and reactive LGL lymphoproliferation occurs most commonly in patients with viral infection such as cytomegalovirus infection and infectious mononucleosis, autoimmune disease or an underlying malignancy [10,22]. In the 2008 WHO classification scheme, T-LGLL is defined as a heterogeneous disorder characterized by a persistent (> 6 months) increase in the number of LGL in the peripheral blood, usually between 2-20 x10^9/L, without a clearly identified cause [23]. In cases with absolute LGL count less than 2 x10^9/L, the diagnosis of T-LGLL could be established if clonal T-cell lymphoproliferation is confirmed, either by TCR gene rearrangement and/or flow cytometry immunophenotyping (aberrancy in T-cell antigen expression or clonal by flow cytometric TCR-Vβ repertoire analysis) [10,24-28]. In most instances, the morphology of the leukemic cells in T-LGLL is indistinguishable from that of the normal LGLs (Fig. 1C), with the exception of extremely rare examples showing markedly pleomorphic nuclei indicating a neoplastic lymphoproliferation (Fig. 1D) [29].

A recent study led by Prof. Kwong YL from Hong Kong characterized 22 Chinese T-LGLL patients in his institution in Hong Kong and found that the most important indication for treatment of their patients was anemia, in contrast to neutropenia in Western patients [30]. Compiling their cases with 88 Asian patients in comparison with 272 Western patients identified from the literature, they found that Asian patients had more frequent anemia (66/110, 60% vs. 113/240, 47%; p=0.044), attributable to a much higher incidence of pure red cell aplasia (PRCA; 52/110, 47% vs. 6/143, 4%; p<0.001) [30]. On the other hand, Western patients presented more frequently with neutropenia (146/235, 62% vs. 33/110, 30%; p<0.001) and splenomegaly (99/246, 40% vs. 16/110, 15%; p<0.001) [30]. Notably, Western patients were about eight to ten times more likely than Asian patients to have rheumatoid arthritis (73/272, 27% vs. 4/106, 4%; p<0.001) and recurrent infections (81/272, 30% vs. 3/107, 3%; p<0.001) [30]. They concluded that different disease mechanisms might be involved in T-LGLL in different populations.

Table 3 summarizes the laboratory and clinical findings of T-LGLL in Taiwan, Hong Kong and the West. Our very recent study of 17 Taiwanese patients with T-LGLL showed a higher mean hemoglobin level (10.5 vs. 8.1 g/dL) and a lower rate of anemia (8/17, 47% vs. 17/22, 77%; p=0.028) as compared to the Chinese patients in Hong Kong; while the frequency of anemia in our patients was similar to that (113/227, 49.8%) of the Western patients (p= 0.988) [10]. Because anemia was not a major problem in our patients and thus bone marrow aspiration/biopsy was performed only in 8 patients. Even so, our cohort of patients showed a lower rate of PRCA as compared to the Hong Kong series (2/8, 25% vs. 17/22, 68%; p=0.035). Interestingly, in our small series of patients, the frequency of PRCA was higher than that (6/143, 4.2%) of the Western patients (p= 0.010). There were no other statistically significant laboratory and clinical parameters between Taiwanese vs. Hong Kong Chinese or Taiwanese vs. Western T-LGLL patients. More studies from East Asian patients are warranted to see if there is a genuine ethnic difference in patients with T-LGLL, particularly in terms of the frequency of anemia and PRCA.

Apart from arising as *de novo* neoplasms, T-LGLL may arise after hematopoietic stem cell or solid organ transplantation [31-38]. Notably, most of the reported cases of T-LGLL after hematopoietic stem cell transplantation are from East Asia. Prof. Kwong's group from Hong Kong recently reported the largest series of 7 such patients who did not have cytopenia, autoimmune phenomenon or organ infiltration, features typical of *de novo* T-LGLL [39]. Excluding 1 patient died from cerebral relapse of the original lymphoma, the remaining 6 patients had remained asymptomatic with stable LGL counts for long periods not requiring any specific treatment. T-LGLL occurring after hematopoietic stem cell transplantation seems to be distinct from *de novo* T-LGLL and may have a different pathogenesis and clinical course.

	Taiwan (n=17)	HK (n=22)	West* (n=272)	P (Taiwan vs. HK)	P (Taiwan vs. West)
Sex					
Male	12	14	125		
Female	5	8	146	0.668	0.050
Age (mean ± SE of the mean, years)	62.1 ± 4.1	52.3 ± 3.2		0.121	
Hemoglobin					
Mean ± SE of the mean (g/dL)	10.5 ± 0.7	8.1 ± 0.7		0.019	
Low(<10 g/dL)	8	17	113	0.028	0.988
Neutrophil count					
Mean ± SE of the mean (x10^9/L)	2.7 ± 0.5	3.4 ± 1.0		0.479	
Low (<1.5x10^9/L)	8	8	146	0.523	0.218
LGL count					
Mean ± SE of the mean (x10^9/L)	4.5 ± 1.2	4.8 ± 0.7		0.523	
High (>2x10^9/L)	11	14	133	0.980	0.110
Platelet count					
Mean ± SE of the mean (x10^9/L)	223 ± 31	204 ± 28		0.989	
Low (<150x10^9/L)	7	5	47	0.337	0.075
Hepatomegaly					
Present	3	5	35		
Absent	7	17	211	0.659	0.169
Splenomegaly					
Present	2	8	99		
Absent	8	14	147	0.335	0.199
Pure red cell aplasia					
Present	2	15	6		
Absent	6	7	137	0.035	0.010
Rheumatoid arthritis					
Present	1	0	73		
Absent	13	22	199	0.203	0.100
Autoimmune phenomena					
Present	0	1	5		
Absent	14	21	267	0.418	0.608

Data from the Western series is based on the report by Prof. Kwong et al [30].

Abbreviation: HK, Hong Kong; SE, standard error.

The statistical analyses of data were performed by student t test or chi square test where appropriate (SPSS, Chicago, IL, USA.)

Table 3. Comparison of T-LGLL in Hong Kong, China, Taiwan and West

In patients with solid organ transplantation clonal T-LGL proliferation seems to be not uncommon. Sabnani et al. found that 71% (10/14) cardiac and 44% (4/9) renal transplant patients had clonal expansion of T-LGL cells but without evidence of either allograft rejection or a viral syndrome. Constitutional symptoms were present in 30% of these patients. Anemia was seen in 75% of renal transplant and 10% of cardiac transplant patients, but none of these patients had significant neutropenia. They believe that this monoclonality is not a true form of post-transplant lymphoproliferative disorder. Constant antigenic stimulus such as a cytomegalovirus reactivation may be the underlying etiology of clonal T-LGL expansion and may contribute to cytopenias and fatigue seen in transplant patients [38].

5. Aggressive NK-cell Leukemia (ANKL)

ANKL is a systemic proliferation of NK-cells, almost always associated with Epstein-Bar virus (EBV) and an aggressive clinical course [40]. This catastrophic disease is observed almost exclusively in Asian patients who are usually very ill on presentation, with pyrexia, jaundice, pancytopenia, skin infiltration, lymphadenopathy and hepatosplenomegaly [40,41]. The most commonly involved sites are peripheral blood, bone marrow, liver and spleen. The leukemic cells may show a wide range of appearance from normal-looking LGL as seen in reactive NK lymphocytosis (Fig. 1E) to atypical (e.g. irregular nuclear foldings, very large size) or immature (e.g. open chromatin, distinct nucleoli) morphological features (Fig. 1F) even in an individual case [42]. The number of neoplastic cells in the peripheral blood and bone marrow can be limited or numerous, from less than 5% to greater than 80% of lymphocytes [42]. Furthermore, there are cases with overlapping features with ENKTL [43,44]. Accordingly, ANKL has also been called aggressive NK-cell lymphoma/leukemia; however, patients with ANKL are younger and the incidence of skin involvement is significantly lower than ENKTL. It is currently unclear whether ANKL is the leukemic counterpart of ENKTL [40].

Phenotypically, the leukemic cells of ANKL in a Japanese series of 22 cases were characterized by the expression of CD2, cytoplasmic CD3, CD56 and HLA-DR with frequent expression of CD7 (14/19 cases, 74%), CD8 and CD16. They did not express surface CD3, CD4, CD5 or CD25 [45]. Interestingly, in a Korean series of 20 cases, CD7 antigen loss was detected in 10 patients (50%) [46]. The Korean investigators claimed that, in conjunction with the cytogenetic findings, this characteristic immunophenotypic finding could serve as a reliable marker for the timely diagnosis in 75% of ANKL [46]. However, there were no statistically significant difference in the clinical or laboratory parameters between the CD7+ and the CD7- ANKL patients. To our knowledge, there are only 2 reports of ANKL from Taiwan, and the leukemic cells in 6 of 7 (86%) cases expressed CD7 [47,48]. No statistically significant difference on CD7 expression was identified between ANKL cases in Taiwan, Japan or Korea (Fishers' exact test).

The great majority of ANKL is associated with EBV-- 85% (11/13) in a Japanese series, 88% (14/16) in a Korean series and 71% (5/7) compiled from the two reports from Taiwan [45,47-49]. The EBV infection in ANKL is an episomal form, indicating a clonal integration into leukemic cells. Prof. Ko et al. compared the clinicopathological characteristics of EBV-negative ANKL patients with those of EBV-positive ANKL patients in Korea and reviewed the literature for reports on EBV-negative ANKL cases. They found that EBV-negative and EBV-positive ANKL patients had similar clinical and pathological characteristics, but EBV-negative patients had a longer survival than EBV-positive patients (11.5 vs. 1.5 months, respectively). EBV-negative patients achieved complete remission, but tumors often relapsed after a short interval, indicating a less aggressive clinical course than EBV-positive ANKL [49].

6. Mature T- and NK/T-cell lymphoma with peripheral blood involvement

The most common T-cell lymphoma with peripheral blood involvement is ATLL and is discussed in the previous chapters. The other T-cell lymphoma with peripheral blood involvement is Sézary syndrome, which is characterized by the triad of erythroderma, generalized lymphadenopathy and the presence of clonally related T-cells with cerebriform nuclei (Sézary cells) in skin, lymph nodes and peripheral blood [50]. Very rarely, PTCL-NOS and ENKTL may progress to bone marrow and peripheral blood involvement, usually in the terminal stage of disease [7,9].

7. Conclusion

In this chapter, we review and analyze various types of T- and NK/T-cell leukemias in the East Asia. Several of these rare neoplasms have not been reported in some East Asian countries yet. Interestingly, there are certain features in some entities, such as T-LGLL, that are distinct from the Western population. More epidemiological, clinicopathological and genetic studies on these rare neoplasms are warranted.

Acknowledgements

The authors are grateful to Prof. Jooryung Huh at Department of Pathology, Asan Medical Center, University of Ulsan College of Medicine, Seoul, Korea and Prof. Ryo Ichinohasama at Division of Hematopathology, Tohoku University Graduate School of Medicine, Sendai, Japan for providing pertinent papers and comments. We thank Prof. Yok-Lam Kwong for providing the photomicrograph of ANKL for figure 1 F.

Author details

Tsung-Hsien Lin[1], Yen-Chuan Hsieh[1,2], Sheng-Tsung Chang[1,3] and Shih-Sung Chuang[1,4]*

*Address all correspondence to: cmh5301@mail.chimei.org.tw

1 Department of Pathology, Chi-Mei Medical Center, Tainan, Taiwan

2 Department of Biological Science and Technology, Chung Hwa University of Medical Technology, Tainan, Taiwan

3 Department of Nursing, National Tainan Institute of Nursing, Tainan, Taiwan

4 Department of Pathology, Taipei Medical University, Taipei, Taiwan

References

[1] Lymphoma Study Group of Japanese Pathologists. The world health organization classification of malignant lymphomas in Japan: incidence of recently recognized entities. Pathol Int. 2000;50:696-702.

[2] Chuang SS, Lin CN, Li CY. Malignant lymphoma in southern Taiwan according to the revised European-American classification of lymphoid neoplasms. Cancer. 2000;89:1586-1592.

[3] Chuang SS. Significant increase in the relative frequency of follicular lymphoma in Taiwan in the early 21st century. J Clin Pathol. 2008;61:879-880.

[4] Yoon SO, Suh C, Lee DH, Chi HS, Park CJ, Jang SS, et al. Distribution of lymphoid neoplasms in the Republic of Korea: analysis of 5318 cases according to the World Health Organization classification. Am J Hematol. 2010;85:760-764.

[5] Miura Y, Fukuhara N, Yamamoto J, Kohata K, Ishizawa K, Ichinohasama R, et al. Clinicopathological features of malignant lymphoma in Japan: the Miyagi Study. Tohoku J Exp Med. 2011;224:151-160.

[6] Swerdlow SH, Campo E, Harris NL, Jaffe ES, Pileri SA, Stein H, et al., ed. WHO classification of tumours of haematopoietic and lymphoid tissues. Lyon: IARC; 2008.

[7] Rezk SA, Huang Q. Extranodal NK/T-cell lymphoma, nasal type extensively involving the bone marrow. Int J Clin Exp Pathol. 2011;4:713-717.

[8] Chan LC, Lam CK, Yeung TC, Chu RW, Ng M, Chow EY, et al. The spectrum of chronic lymphoproliferative disorders in Hong Kong. A prospective study. Leukemia. 1997;11:1964-1972.

[9]   Chang ST, Hsieh YC, Kuo SY, Lu CL, Chu JS, Chuang SS. The spectrum of T-cell and natural killer/T-cell neoplasms with leukaemic presentation in a single institution in Taiwan. Int J Lab Hematol. 2012;34:422-426.

[10] Hsieh YC, Chang ST, Huang WT, Kuo SY, Chiang TA, Chuang SS. A Comparative Study of Flow Cytometric T-cell Receptor Vβ Repertoire and T-cell Receptor Gene Rearrangement in the Diagnosis of Large Granular Lymphocytic Lymphoprolifera- tion. Int J Lab Hematol. 2012 in press.

[11] Suzumiya J, Ohshima K, Kikuchi M, Takeshita M, Akamatsu M, Tashiro K. Terminal deoxynucleotidyl transferase staining of malignant lymphomas in paraffin sections: a useful method for the diagnosis of lymphoblastic lymphoma. J Pathol. 1997;182:86-91.

[12] Pui CH, Hancock ML, Head DR, Rivera GK, Look AT, Sandlund JT, et al. Clinical sig- nificance of CD34 expression in childhood acute lymphoblastic leukemia. Blood. 1993;82:889-894.

[13] Robertson PB, Neiman RS, Worapongpaiboon S, John K, Orazi A. 013 (CD99) positiv- ity in hematologic proliferations correlates with TdT positivity. Mod Pathol. 1997;10:277-282.

[14] Terada T. TDT (-), KIT (+), CD34 (+), CD99 (+) precursor T lymphoblastic leukemia/ lymphoma. Int J Clin Exp Pathol. 2012;5:167-170.

[15] Hoelzer D, Gokbuget N. T-cell lymphoblastic lymphoma and T-cell acute lympho- blastic leukemia: a separate entity? Clin Lymphoma Myeloma. 2009;9 Suppl 3:S214-221.

[16] Matutes E, Brito-Babapulle V, Swansbury J, Ellis J, Morilla R, Dearden C, et al. Clini- cal and laboratory features of 78 cases of T-prolymphocytic leukemia. Blood. 1991;78:3269-3274.

[17] Kameoka J, Takahashi N, Noji H, Murai K, Tajima K, Kameoka Y, et al. T-cell pro- lymphocytic leukemia in Japan: is it a variant? Int J Hematol. 2012;95:660-667.

[18] Kojima K, Kobayashi H, Imoto S, Nakagawa T, Matsui T, Kawachi Y, et al. 14q11 ab- normality and trisomy 8q are not common in Japanese T-cell prolymphocytic leuke- mia. Int J Hematol. 1998;68:291-296.

[19] Yokohama A, Saitoh A, Nakahashi H, Mitsui T, Koiso H, Kim Y, et al. TCL1A gene involvement in T-cell prolymphocytic leukemia in Japanese patients. Int J Hematol. 2102;95:77-85.

[20] Jeong KH, Lew BL, Sim WY. Generalized leukaemia cutis from a small cell variant of T-cell prolymphocytic leukaemia presenting with exfoliative dermatitis. Acta Derm Venereol. 2009;89:509-512.

[21] Sokol L, Loughran TP, Jr. Large granular lymphocyte leukemia. Oncologist. 2006;11:263-273.

[22] O'Malley DP. T-cell large granular leukemia and related proliferations. Am J Clin Pathol. 2007;127:850-859.

[23] Chan WC, Foucar K, Morice WG, Catovsky D. T-cell large granular lymphocytic leukemia. In: Swerdlow SH, Campo E, Harris NL, Jaffe ES, Pileri SA, Stein H, et al., ed. WHO classification of tumours of haemtopoietic and lymphoid tissues. Lyon: IARC; 2008:272-273.

[24] Lima M, Almeida J, Santos AH, dos Anjos Teixeira M, Alguero MC, Queirós ML, et al. Immunophenotypic analysis of the TCR-Vbeta repertoire in 98 persistent expansions of CD3(+)/TCR-alphabeta(+) large granular lymphocytes: utility in assessing clonality and insights into the pathogenesis of the disease. Am J Pathol. 2001;159:1861-1868.

[25] Morice WG, Kimlinger T, Katzmann JA, Lust JA, Heimgartner PJ, Halling KC, et al. Flow cytometric assessment of TCR-Vbeta expression in the evaluation of peripheral blood involvement by T-cell lymphoproliferative disorders: a comparison with conventional T-cell immunophenotyping and molecular genetic techniques. Am J Clin Pathol. 2004;121:373-383.

[26] Feng B, Jorgensen JL, Hu Y, Medeiros LJ, Wang SA. TCR-Vbeta flow cytometric analysis of peripheral blood for assessing clonality and disease burden in patients with T cell large granular lymphocyte leukaemia. J Clin Pathol. 2010;63:141-146.

[27] Bareau B, Rey J, Hamidou M, Donadieu J, Morcet J, Reman O, et al. Analysis of a French cohort of patients with large granular lymphocyte leukemia: a report on 229 cases. Haematologica. 2010;95:1534-1541.

[28] Lamy T, Loughran TP, Jr. How I treat LGL leukemia. Blood. 2011;117:2764-2774.

[29] Chang ST, Hsieh YC, Chen CH, Tsao CJ, Chuang SS. T-cell large granular lymphocytic leukemia with pleomorphic nuclei and colonic infiltration with chronic diarrhea. Leuk Lymphoma. 2010;51:2132-2134.

[30] Kwong YL, Au WY, Leung AY, Tse EW. T-cell large granular lymphocyte leukemia: an Asian perspective. Ann Hematol. 2010;89:331-339.

[31] Gentile TC, Hadlock KG, Uner AH, Delal B, Squiers E, Crowley S, et al. Large granular lymphocyte leukaemia occurring after renal transplantation. Br J Haematol. 1998;101:507-512.

[32] Au WY, Lam CC, Lie AK, Pang A, Kwong YL. T-cell large granular lymphocyte leukemia of donor origin after allogeneic bone marrow transplantation. Am J Clin Pathol. 2003;120:626-630.

[33] Lau LG, Tan LK, Salto-Tellez M, Koay ES, Liu TC. T-cell post-transplant lymphoproliferative disorder after hematopoietic stem cell transplantation: another case and a review of the literature. Bone Marrow Transplant. 2004;34:821-822.

[34] Narumi H, Kojima K, Matsuo Y, Shikata H, Sekiya K, Niiya T, et al. T-cell large gran-
      ular lymphocytic leukemia occurring after autologous peripheral blood stem cell
      transplantation. Bone Marrow Transplant. 2004;33:99-101.

[35] Chang H, Kamel-Reid S, Hussain N, Lipton J, Messner HA. T-cell large granular lym-
      phocytic leukemia of donor origin occurring after allogeneic bone marrow transplan-
      tation for B-cell lymphoproliferative disorders. Am J Clin Pathol. 2005;123:196-199.

[36] Sabnani I, Zucker MJ, Tsang P, Palekar S. Clonal T-large granular lymphocyte prolif-
      eration in solid organ transplant recipients. Transplant Proc. 2006;38:3437-3440.

[37] Kusumoto S, Mori S, Nosaka K, Morita-Hoshi Y, Onishi Y, Kim SW, et al. T-cell large
      granular lymphocyte leukemia of donor origin after cord blood transplantation. Clin
      Lymphoma Myeloma. 2007;7:475-479.

[38] Nann-Rutti S, Tzankov A, Cantoni N, Morita-Hoshi Y, Onishi Y, Kim SW, et al. Large
      Granular Lymphocyte Expansion after Allogeneic Hematopoietic Stem Cell Trans-
      plant is Associated with a Cytomegalovirus Reactivation and Shows an Indolent
      Outcome. Biol Blood Marrow Transplant. 2012;18:1765-1770 [Epub ahead of print].

[39] Gill H, Ip AH, Leung R, So JC, Pang AW, Tse E, et al. Indolent T-cell large granular
      lymphocyte leukaemia after haematopoietic SCT: a clinicopathologic and molecular
      analysis. 2012;47:952-956.

[40] Chan JKC, Jaffe ES, Ralfkiaer E, Ko Y-H. Aggressive NK/T-cell lymphoma. In: Swer-
      dlow SH, Campo E, Harris NL, Jaffe ES, Pileri SA, Stein H, et al., ed. WHO classifica-
      tion of tumours of haemtopoietic and lymphoid tissues. Lyon: IARC; 2008:276-277.

[41] Kwong YL. Natural killer-cell malignancies: diagnosis and treatment. Leukemia.
      2005;19:2186-2194.

[42] Cheuk W, Chan J, K.C. Chapter 28. NK-cell neoplasms. In: Jaffe ES, Harris NL, Vardi-
      man JW, Campo E, Arber DA, ed. Hematopathology. St. Louis: Saunders;
      2011:473-491.

[43] Kim SH, Ko WT, Suh MK, Ha GY, Kim JR. A case of aggressive NK/T-cell lympho-
      ma/leukemia with cutaneous involvement in adolescence. Ann Dermatol (Seoul).
      2008;20:77-81.

[44] Chan JKC, Quintanilla-Martinez L, Ferry JA, Peh S-C. Extranodal NK/T-cell lympho-
      ma, nasal type. In: Swerdlow SH, Campo E, Harris NL, Jaffe ES, Pileri SA, Stein H, et
      al., ed. WHO classification of tumours of haemtopoietic and lymphoid tissues. Lyon:
      IARC; 2008:285-288.

[45] Suzuki R, Suzumiya J, Nakamura S, Aoki S, Notoya A, Ozaki S, et al. Aggressive nat-
      ural killer-cell leukemia revisited: large granular lymphocyte leukemia of cytotoxic
      NK cells. Leukemia. 2004;18:763-770.

[46] Yoo EH, Kim HJ, Lee ST, Kim WS, Kim SH. Frequent CD7 antigen loss in aggressive natural killer-cell leukemia: a useful diagnostic marker. Korean J Lab Med. 2009;29:491-496.

[47] Chou WC, Chiang IP, Tang JL, Su IJ, Huang SY, Chen YC, et al. Clonal disease of natural killer large granular lymphocytes in Taiwan. Br J Haematol. 1998;103:1124-1128.

[48] Lee PS, Hwang WS. Aggressive natural killer cell lymphoma/leukemia. Chi Med J (Taipei). 2002;65:622-626.

[49] Ko YH, Park S, Kim K, Kim SJ, Kim WS. Aggressive natural killer cell leukemia: is Epstein-Barr virus negativity an indicator of a favorable prognosis? Acta Haematol. 2008;120:199-206.

[50] Ralfkiaer E, Willemze R, Whittaker SJ. Sézary syndrome. In: Swerdlow SH, Campo E, Harris NL, Jaffe ES, Pileri SA, Stein H, et al., ed. WHO classification of tumours of haemtopoietic and lymphoid tissues. Lyon: IARC; 2008:299.

Chapter 3

Pleiotropic Functions of
HTLV-1 Tax Contribute to Cellular Transformation

Kendle Pryor and Susan J. Marriott

Additional information is available at the end of the chapter

1. Introduction

Human T cell leukemia virus type-1 (HTLV-1) is the only retrovirus known to be the etiologic agent of a human cancer, adult T-cell leukemia/lymphoma (ATLL), a highly aggressive cancer of mature T cells. Epidemiological reports suggest that 10 to 20 million people throughout the world are infected with HTLV-1, which is endemic in parts of sub-Saharan Africa, the Caribbean, Japan, and South America [1]. HTLV-1 encodes a regulatory protein, Tax, which is essential for virus replication and plays a significant role in the oncogenic potential of HTLV-1. This chapter will summarize the effects of Tax on cellular processes including transcription, cell cycle checkpoints, and DNA repair, and will discuss how these activities may contribute to its transforming potential.

2. HTLV-1 epidemiology and pathogenesis

HTLV-1 is a type C, complex, enveloped retrovirus belonging to the family *Retroviridae* and the genus deltaretrovirus. This genus includes three additional HTLV members (HTLV-2, -3, and -4), and two non-human members, bovine leukemia virus (BLV), and simian T cell leukemia virus (STLV). HTLV-1 was originally isolated from a patient diagnosed with cutaneous T cell lymphoma, and was subsequently shown to be the causative agent of ATLL [2-4]. HTLV-1 is also recognized as the etiologic agent of a neurodegenerative disease, tropical spastic paraparesis/HTLV-1 associated myelopathy (TSP/HAM), that affects the central nervous system [5,6]. The route of HTLV-1 transmission influences its pathogenesis. Sexual transmission, which occurs most efficiently from males to females, IV drug use, and blood transfusions are typically associated with the development of TSP/HAM, whereas the most common route of transmission, mother to child, is preferentially associated with the development of ATLL [7-12].

ATLL, a rapidly progressing cancer of mature CD4$^+$ T cells, has been classified into four clinical subtypes:, smoldering, chronic, lymphoma, and acute [13]. Leukemic cells from ATLL patients have a phenotype of CD2$^+$, CD3$^+$, CD4$^+$, CD8$^-$, and HLA-DR$^+$, express high levels of interleukin 2 (IL-2) and its receptor (IL-2R), and frequently have lobulated nuclei, causing them to be referred to as flower cells. Interestingly, these cells are only moderately responsive to IL-2, and HTLV-1 infected T cells proliferate continuously in the absence of exogenous IL-2, a characteristic associated with late stage T-cell transformation [14]. Other members of the deltaretrovirus family have also been linked to proliferative diseases. For instance, sheep infected with BLV develop B-cell leukemia/lymphoma, and the simian counterpart of HTLV-1, STLV-1, induces an ATLL like disease in African green monkeys [15,16]. In contrast, HTLV-2 has not been definitively linked to human cancer and the disease potentials of the newly discovered HTLV-3 and -4 viruses remain unknown [17,18].

2.1. HTLV-1 genome

The HTLV-1 proviral genome is approximately 9 kb in length including flanking long terminal repeats (LTR) composed of U3, R, and U5 regions. HTLV-1 encodes structural (*gag*, *env*) and enzymatic (*pro*, *pol*) genes typical of all retroviruses. In addition, a highly conserved pX region located near the 3' LTR, encodes four open reading frames (ORFs) that produce regulatory proteins [19,20]. ORF I encodes p12, which undergoes proteolytic cleavage to generate p8. Alternative splicing of ORF II produces the p13 and p30 proteins. Analysis of full-length infectious molecular clones of HTLV-1 containing mutations in p12, p13, and/or p30 in a rabbit infection model demonstrated an important role for these viral accessory proteins in establishing and maintaining viral persistence [21-26]. ORFs III and IV produce doubly spliced mRNA encoding Rex and the viral oncoprotein Tax, respectively. These proteins differentially regulate transcription, which is essential for viral replication [26-29]. Rex is a 27 kDa protein that regulates post-transcriptional viral gene expression by transporting unspliced mRNA from the nucleus to the cytoplasm and increases viral RNA stability, potentially influencing latent and productive phases of the virus life cycle [26,29]. Tax is a potent transcriptional regulator of viral and cellular gene expression and modulates cellular protein function. Unlike Tax, HBZ is transcribed from the antisense strand of the proviral genome and appears to be constitutively expressed in HTLV-1-infected and ATLL cells [30]. HBZ promotes the proliferation of human T cells and may play an important role in maintaining malignant transformation of HTLV-1 infected T cells [31]. The mechanisms of Tax-mediated cellular transformation will be discussed below.

2.2. Transformation by HTLV-1

Multiple studies have demonstrated that Tax is sufficient for cellular transformation and is important for HTLV-1 mediated tumorigenesis [32-38]. Acute transforming retroviruses rapidly induce tumors by expressing a viral oncogene [39]. In contrast, chronic transforming retroviruses induce tumors at a much slower rate by aberrantly regulating genes upstream or downstream of the proviral insertion site [40]. Neither of these models explains HTLV-1 mediated transformation since no cellular homologue of Tax has been identified and HTLV-1 integration is random. The oncogenic potential of Tax has been extensively characterized in rodent fibroblast cell culture systems, transgenic mouse models, and immortalization and transformation studies in primary human T cells.

One of the first studies to show that Tax could independently transform human T cells used a transformation–defective but replication competent *herpes saimiri* vector encoding Tax to infect primary cord blood lymphocytes [32]. The transformed T cells were CD4+/CD8- and expressed high levels of IL-2R, resulting in clonally expanded cell populations similar to ATLL cells. Deletion of the Tax gene in this vector eliminated its transforming potential [32]. In addition, a replication defective HTLV-1 provirus isolated from leukemic cells of an ATLL patient expressed Tax and promoted loss of contact inhibition and anchorage-independent growth in rodent fibroblasts [37]. Mutation of the Tax gene in this proviral vector reduced tumor formation in nude mice, suggesting that Tax is required for the transforming potential of HTLV-1. Loss of Tax expression in HTLV-1-transformed Rat-1 cells resulted in an inability to form tumors and restoring Tax expression restored the tumorigenic potential of these cells, indicating that Tax is required to establish transformation [38]. In combination with *ras*, Tax is sufficient to transform primary rat embryo fibroblast cells in culture and to induce tumors in nude mice. Tax alone can transform Rat-2 cells and induce tumors in athymic mice [41]. These studies demonstrated that HTLV-1 is a transforming retrovirus with a broad transforming potential not limited to primary T cells, and that Tax is necessary and sufficient to transform cells *in vitro* and induce tumor formation *in vivo*.

3. Characterization of Tax-induced tumors in transgenic mouse models

To determine whether Tax plays a role in HTLV-1 induced leukemia/lymphoma, first generation transgenic mouse models expressing Tax under the control of the HTLV-1 LTR were developed, resulting in broad expression of Tax in tissues including thymus, lung, and brain [35]. Interestingly, these mice developed neurofibromas and mesenchymal tumors with visual tumors on the ears, feet, and tail, instead of T cell derived lymphoid tumors, indicating that Tax expression driven by the HTLV-1 promoter leads to neurotropic associated tumor development in this model [35]. To generate a mouse model that more closely recapitulates ATLL, second generation transgenic mice expressed Tax under control of the human granzyme B (GzmB) promoter, which limits transgene expression to CD4+ and CD8+ T lymphocytes (T), natural killer (NK), and lymphokine-activated killer cells [42]. These GzmB-Tax mice developed T-cell lymphomas that expressed high levels of nuclear factor kappa B (NF-κB) [42]. Antisense inhibition of NF-κB expression resulted in tumor regression suggesting that Tax-dependent tumor formation and regression correlate with NF-κB expression [43]. Although GzmB-Tax mice presented with hepatosplenomegaly similar to ATLL patients, they developed large granulocytic leukemia (LGL) indicative of infiltrating neutrophils, basophils, and eosinophils [42]. LGL tumor cells exhibited antibody-dependent cellular cytotoxicity, a primary function of NK-cells, and did not express T-lymphocyte markers, thus these tumors were derived from malignant NK cells [42,44]. Although GzmB-Tax mice did not develop T-cell leukemia/lymphoma, this model demonstrated that limiting Tax expression to the lymphoid compartment could drive lymphomagenesis.

Third generation transgenic mice expressed Tax under the control of the Lck promoter, which restricts expression to developing thymocytes [45]. At 10 months of age, Lck-Tax transgenic mice developed swollen and enlarged spleens, livers, and lymph nodes, recapitulating clinical features observed in patients with ATLL, and presented with large mesenteric tumors [45]. These mice displayed skin ulcerations involving infiltration of leukemic cells in to the dermis, and lymphoma cells from these tumors had a "flower-like" morphology consistent with ATLL cells [45]. Engraftment of these tumor cells into SCID mice led to the development of an aggressive and rapidly progressing leukemia resulting in death within 28 days, similar to the aggressive nature of ATLL [45]. Although Lck-Tax mice recapitulate the clinical features of ATLL, isolated tumor cells were CD25$^+$, CD44$^+$, CD69$^+$, but CD4$^-$/CD8$^-$ double negative, indicating that the lymphomas were derived from malignant transformation of immature T cells [45]. In this model restriction of Tax expression to the T cell compartment produced transgenic mice having clinical features of ATLL however, the absence of CD4$^+$ lymphomas and continued expression of Tax in the tumor cells does not precisely model ATLL in these mice.

HTLV-1 humanized SCID mice (HTLV-1-Hu-SCID) were generated by reconstituting hematopoiesis in non-obese SCID mice using human CD34$^+$ hematopoietic progenitor stem cells (HPSCs) infected with HTLV-1 [46]. Within 12-20 weeks of reconstitution, the Hu-SCID mice developed CD4$^+$ T cell lymphomas with clinical and histopathological features similar to ATLL and Lck-Tax transgenic mice [45,46]. Isolated tumor cells expressed HTLV-1 Gag, CD25, CD4, and CD8 proteins, demonstrating that the tumor cells originated from malignant transformation of mature T cells [46]. Additionally, Hu-SCID mice generated using HPSCs infected with a lentiviral vector expressing Tax (Tax-Hu-SCID) developed monoclonal CD4$^+$ tumors suggesting that reconstituting mice with a human hematopoietic system drives Tax-mediated lymphomagenesis of mature T cells [46]. The HTLV-1 infected Hu-SCID mouse model provides a promising tool with which to assess the development and progression of HTLV-1-induced CD4$^+$ T cell lymphomas.

4. Molecular mechanisms of Tax mediated transformation

4.1. Regulation of CREB and NFκB pathways by Tax

Since multiple studies have shown that Tax is sufficient for cellular transformation and is important for HTLV-1 mediated lymphomagenesis [32-38] much effort has been invested into understanding the molecular mechanisms that drive Tax-mediated transformation and tumorigenesis. Microarray analysis of HTLV-1 infected and Tax transfected cells demonstrated genome-wide changes in cellular gene expression patterns including changes in the expression of genes that control proliferation, cell cycle checkpoints, apoptosis, and transcription, suggesting potential pathways through which Tax might function to modulate normal cellular responses [47,48]. Extensive mutational analysis of Tax revealed the presence of a nuclear localization signal, nuclear export signal, and activation domains specific for the NF-κB and cAMP-responsive element binding protein (CREB) pathways [49-51]. Tax does not bind DNA but, interacts with cellular proteins to modulate at least three major transcription factor pathways NF-κB, CREB, and serum response factor (SRF) pathways, of which the CREB and NF-κB pathways have been most extensively studied [52-62] and shown to be essential for Tax-mediated transformation.

Modulation of the CREB pathway by Tax is important for transcriptional activation of the HTLV-1 promoter (LTR). The HTLV-1 LTR contains three non-palindromic 21-bp repeats called Tax responsive elements (TRE). Each TRE contains a core CRE sequence flanked by GC-rich sequences, which are required for Tax-mediated transactivation. Under normal physiological conditions, CREB activation is initiated by growth factor stimulated phosphorylation of the kinase inducible domain (KID) of CREB followed by CREB dimerization and recruitment of the CREB binding protein (CBP) through its KID interaction KIX domain [63,64]. The CBP-CREB complex then binds to palindromic CREs to activate transcription of CREB-dependent genes. In Tax expressing cells, Tax interacts with CREB to enhance CREB dimerization and selectively increase the binding affinity of CREB for the viral TRE, which is mediated by the flanking GC rich regions [65-67]. Tax also interacts with the KIX domain of CBP and its homologue p300 to enhance their recruitment to the Tax-CREB-TRE ternary complex, thereby stabilizing the complex and activating viral gene expression in the absence of CREB phosphorylation [67-71]. Thus, Tax can bypass cAMP signaling mediated activation of CREB and induce preferential binding of CREB to the viral LTR rather than to cellular CREs. These results emphasize the importance of the CREB pathway for viral gene expression [54,66,70,70,71,71]

Tax regulation of cellular gene expression through the NF-κB pathway results in cell proliferation, resistance to apoptosis, and maintenance of malignant transformation. In a resting cell, NF-κB is sequestered in the cytoplasm in an inactive complex with inhibitor of kappa B (IκB), which prevents activation of NF-κB -dependent genes [72]. External growth factor stimulation initiates a signaling cascade that induces phosphorylation of IκB by IκB kinase (IKK), resulting in ubiquitination, and subsequent degradation of IκB, which then releases NF-κB to translocate to the nucleus and activate NF-κB-dependent gene expression. Tax disrupts NF-κB regulation by several mechanisms. First, cytoplasmic Tax increases phosphorylation and subsequent degradation of IκBα by forming a ternary complex containing NF-κB essential modulator (NEMO), IKKγ, Tax, and PP2A that blocks deactivation of IKK [73-76]. Constitutively active IKK results in persistent IκB degradation and translocation of NF-κB to the nucleus. Second, nuclear Tax interacts with NF-κB on promoters resulting in constitutive activation of NF-κB dependent genes [77,78]. Persistent degradation of IκB and constitutive activation of NF-κB dependent genes leads to persistent activation of the NF-κB pathway in HTLV-1 infected, and Tax-expressing cells [79]. Upregulation of NF-κB-dependent genes including, but not limited to key T cell activators (IL-2, high affinity IL-2R alpha subunit, and IL-15) is required for immortalization and survival of HTLV-1 transformed cells, setting the stage for neoplastic conversion of a normal T cell [53,60,80]

4.2. CREB and NF-κB pathways in Tax-mediated transformation

A Tax mutant (M47) that is defective for activation of CREB-dependent genes did not induce loss of contact inhibition or anchorage independent growth in Rat 2 cells and failed to induce tumors in nude mice [36], suggesting that activation of the CREB pathway is required to establish Tax-induced tumors. In the same study, a Tax mutant (M22) that is defective for NF-κB activation did transform Rat 2 cells in vitro and induce tumors in athymic mice similar to wild-type Tax, indicating that NF-κB activation is not required to initiate Tax-mediated tumorigenesis [36]. In a different study, a *herpesvirus saimiri* vector carrying the Tax S258A mutant that is defective for NF-κB activity, retained the ability to immortalize PBMCs, which is a prerequisite for transformation [81]. However, a Tax mutant (M319) that fails to activate CREB dependent genes comparable to Tax M47 induced anchorage independent growth in Rat-1 cells and tumor formation in nude mice, suggesting that CREB activation is not required for transformation [82]. Differences between the effect of CREB mutants in this study and the previous study may be due to differences in the specific cell lines and Tax mutants used in the studies. However, since NF-κB mutants retained transforming ability in both studies, and since ablation of NF-κB expression in established Tax tumors led to tumor regression, there is strong evidence that NF-κB is required for tumor maintenance, but not for tumor induction [43]. Analysis of the roles of the CREB and NF-κB pathways in Tax mediated transformation reveal complex effects on tumor initiation, and maintenance. Taken together, the effects of Tax on, NF-κB, IκB, CREB, and CBP/p300 appear to commit a normal cell to a highly proliferative state, setting the stage for the development of ATLL (Figure 1).

5. Effect of Tax on genome stability

5.1. Disruption of DNA repair pathways by Tax

DNA repair and cell cycle progression are tightly linked and involve multiple overlapping pathways that ensure error-free inheritance of genetic material. If a cell incurs extensive DNA damage that cannot be repaired, it will undergo apoptosis or enter a state of replicative senescence. Tax disrupts DNA repair by modulating the functions of key DNA repair enzymes and disrupting the DNA damage response (DDR), resulting in an increased mutation frequency in Tax-expressing cells [83,84]. Cellular DNA damage is repaired by four functionally overlapping pathways that respond to different types of DNA alterations; mismatch repair (MMR) base excision repair (BER), nucleotide excision repair (NER), and double strand break repair (DSBR) [85]. The suppression or disruption of BER, NER or DSBR by Tax appears to contribute to its cellular transformation activity.

BER is initiated by a glycosylase that recognizes helical distortions and flips out the base promoting recruitment of a major repair enzyme, DNA polymerase beta (pol β) [86,87]. Tax has been shown to repress pol β transcription [88,89]. The decreased availability of pol β would reduce the efficient repair of DNA lesions that arise from reactive oxygen species and depurination events consistent with increased mutagenesis of the host genome.

The NER pathway preserves genome stability by scanning for and repairing UV- and chemically-induced bulky adducts [85]. Proliferating cell nuclear antigen (PCNA) is a trimeric sliding clamp that assists in DNA synthesis during DNA replication and repair, by increasing the processivity of DNA polymerase delta (pol δ) to fill in the gap after lesion excision [85,90,91]. In the presence of DNA lesions, elevated levels of p21[Cip1/waf1] interact with PCNA to block DNA replication without blocking PCNA-dependent DNA repair [92]. Tax activates PCNA gene expression [93], which may allow Tax-expressing cells to overwhelm the p21[Cip1/waf1]-induced replication block and continue DNA replication in the presence of damage, resulting in misincorporation of DNA nucleotides [94,95]. Thus, Tax appears to suppress NER and promote genome instability by increasing the cellular mutation rate.

Unlike NER and BER, less is known about effects of Tax on the DSBR pathway. Double strand DNA breaks (DSBs) are sensed by ataxia telangiectasia mutated (ATM) kinase, which phosphorylates downstream DNA damage checkpoint regulators such as H2AX, Chk2, p53, Nbs1 and MDC1 that function together to arrest the cell cycle and repair DNA [96]. ATM signaling also promotes the recruitment of Ku70 and Ku80 hetereodimers to free DNA ends to facilitate DNA end joining. Tax has been shown to repress Ku80 gene expression, which may impact the cell's ability to recognize and repair free DNA ends [97,98]. In addition, the phosphorylation of ATM targets (H2AX, Chk2 and Nsb1) and ATM autophosphorylation is reduced in Tax-expressing cells, which attenuates the DDR, causing these cells to be released from the S-phase checkpoint while DSBs remain [99-101]. Cells that undergo mitosis in the presence of DSBs frequently form micronuclei (MN), which are markers of genome instability and interestingly, Tax-expressing cells exhibit significantly more micronuclei than control cells [101]. Since, the response to DNA damage and the initiation of DNA repair are tightly linked, the effect of Tax on early cellular processes such as ATM-mediated DNA damage signaling, translates to defects in later processes including cell cycle checkpoints and DNA repair, creating an environment that promotes cellular transformation as shown in Figure 1.

5.2. Impact of Tax on cell cycle regulation

Under normal conditions, eukaryotic cells undergo growth and division resulting in the passage of genetic information, which is essential for survival. Eukaryotic cell division is controlled by four distinct phases: cell growth (G_1, and G_2), DNA synthesis (S), and mitosis (M). Critical cell cycle checkpoints (G_1/S, G_2/M, and M) can be activated to block cell cycle progression and ensure accurate DNA replication and chromosome distribution. Specific complexes containing cyclins, cyclin-dependent kinases (CDK), CDK inhibitors (CKIs), and tumor suppressor proteins work together to maintain genome integrity and prevent uncontrolled proliferation.

Prior to entering G_1, mitogenic stimulation increases the levels of type D (D1, D2, and D3) and E (E1, E2) cyclins. During early G_1 of a normal cell, active D-CDK4/6 complexes phosphorylate the tumor suppressor retinoblastoma (Rb), allowing release of transcription factor E2F and subsequent activation of S phase genes [102]. At this stage, cells are committed to entering S phase where the E-CDK2 complex phosphorylates substrates needed for S phase. Tax expression accelerates progression through G_1 by activating the transcription of genes encoding D cyclins, which directly interact with D-CDK4/6 to enhance Rb phosphorylation [103-105]. Following its release and translocation to the nucleus, E2F interacts with Tax to transcribe E2F-dependent S phase genes [103]. These transcriptional effects, and modulation of CDK complexes propel Tax-expressing cells through G_1 and force early entry into S phase [104-106].

During the transition from G_1 to S, cells pass through a checkpoint regulated by p53. The tumor suppressor p53 protects cells from transformation by activating the expression of cell cycle control proteins [107] that mediate cell cycle arrest or apoptosis in response to various cellular stresses, including DNA damage. In the presence of DNA damage, p53 arrests the cell cycle by activating the CKI p21$^{wafl/cip1}$, which binds and inactivates CDK2. Therefore, overexpression of p21$^{wafl/cip1}$ induces cell cycle arrest and prevents progression into S-phase until DNA is repaired. p21$^{wafl/cip1}$ also binds to and stabilizes the cyclin D-CDK4/6 complex, leading to increased kinase activity and cell cycle progression, which is consistent with p21$^{wafl/cip1}$ overexpression in Tax-transfected and HTLV-1 transformed cells [108,109]. In addition, Tax-expressing cells display a shortened G_1 phase followed by early S-phase entry, suggesting that the G_1/S checkpoint is deregulated to avoid p21$^{wafl/cip1}$ induced cell cycle arrest [110]. Tax mediated overexpression of p21$^{wafl/cip1}$ may contribute to transformation by accelerating the progression of cells through G_1 and disrupting the DNA damage-induced G_1/S checkpoint [108,111,112].

Further disruption of the G_1/S checkpoint occurs by Tax-mediated inactivation of p53. Tax and p53 have been shown to directly compete for binding to the coactivator CBP/p300, thus p53-dependent transcription could be compromised in Tax-expressing cells [113-115]. Tax has also been shown to suppress p53 function by inducing hyperphosphorylation of p53 at Ser$_{15}$ and Ser$_{392}$, preventing p53 from interacting with the basal transcription machinery [116,117]. In supporting studies, Tax mutants defective in NF-κB activation failed to suppress p53-mediated transcription [117,118]. Thus, the transcriptional activity of Tax affects p53 regulation of cell cycle checkpoints, DDR and DNA repair, thereby altering the cell's response to internal and external stress stimuli.

Although p53 and p21$^{wafl/cip1}$ prevent unchecked proliferation and genome stability, additional CKIs prevent replication of damaged DNA by inhibiting cyclin-CDK interactions [119,120]. Tax regulates the function of cyclin-CDK complexes by disrupting the inhibitory activities of CDK4 (INK4) inhibitors p15^{INK4b} (p15), p16^{INK4a} (p16), p18^{INK4c} (p18), and p19^{INK4d} (p19), which share overlapping functions to regulate G_1 entry and progression. Before entering G_1 external anti-growth factors such as transforming growth beta (TGF-β) can stimulate cell cycle exit by inducing the binding of p15 to D-CDK4/6 complexes, thereby promoting the degradation of D cyclins [121]. Because a decrease in active D-CDK4/6 complexes prevents cell cycle progression, cellular mechanisms to promote cyclin D overexpression could antagonize p15-mediated arrest. Specifically, the overexpression of D-cyclins and p21$^{wafl/cip1}$ in Tax expressing cells correlates with increased cell proliferation, consistent with cell cycle progression in the presence of genome instability. Tax also binds to p16 and suppresses its inhibitory function by allowing cyclin D1 to form active complexes with CDK4/6. Inhibition of p15 and p16 by Tax increases the pool of active D-CDK4/6 complexes resulting in continuous Rb phosphorylation and leading to S phase entry [122,123]. Lastly, Tax represses transcription of p18^{INK4c}, and p19^{INK4d}, again linking Tax-mediated transcription with cell cycle deregulation [112,122-125]. Cumulative effects of Tax on the G_1 and the G_1/S checkpoints contribute to Tax mediated transformation by continuously promoting cell growth and proliferation in the absence of growth factors.

During S phase, cyclin A-CDK2 begins to accumulate after the G_1/S transition, and is required both to complete S phase and to enter and exit from M phase. HTLV-1 infected cells express low levels of cyclin A because Tax represses cyclin A transcription in a CREB-ATF-dependent manner [126]. Reduced cyclin A levels also promote early egress from mitosis and disrupt the G_2/M checkpoint, producing the types of chromosomal abnormalities observed in ATLL and HTLV-1 transformed cells [127-135].

When cells sense DNA-damage prior to mitosis the G_2/M DNA-damage checkpoint is activated through two DNA damage sensors ATM and ATR, which phosphorylate downstream effectors such as p53, and checkpoint kinases 1 and 2 (Chk1 and Chk2). These downstream effectors phosphorylate downstream substrates to induce cell cycle arrest. Following DNA damage, phosphorylation of Cdc25A by Chk1 targets it for proteasomal degradation, thereby inhibiting activation of the Cdk1/2 complex, which is required to progress through the S and G_2/M checkpoints. Chk1 also phosphorylates p53 and CDC25A/C to induce G_1 and G_2/M arrest, respectively. In response to gamma irradiation, Tax interacts with Chk1 and inhibits its kinase activity, thereby disrupting the G_1 and G_2/M checkpoints and allowing cells to proceed to mitosis in the presence of DNA damage [136]. Interestingly, Tax prevents the release of Chk2 from chromatin after activation by ATM/ATR, thereby preventing phosphorylation of downstream effectors like p53 [137]. Tax disruption of cell cycle regulation and abrogation of the DNA damage response contributes to the proliferation of cells containing DNA damage.

After transiting the G_2/M checkpoint, the cell encounters one last critical checkpoint known as the mitotic spindle checkpoint (MSC). The MSC regulates cell cycle transition from metaphase to anaphase, and its disruption is associated with altered chromosome structures and numbers [138]. HTLV-1 infected/transformed cells and ATLL cells display chromosomal abnormalities including deletions, insertions, rearrangements and translocations, suggesting that Tax disrupts the MSC [127-135,139,140]. The direct interaction of Tax with MAD-1 and APC interferes with proper chromosome alignment along the metaphase plate resulting in the potential loss or gain of genetic material and early exit from mitosis [141,142]. The intimate linkage between the DDR and DNA repair expands the effects of Tax on normal cell proliferation by targeting cell modulators, such as p53, that function in multiple cellular processes.

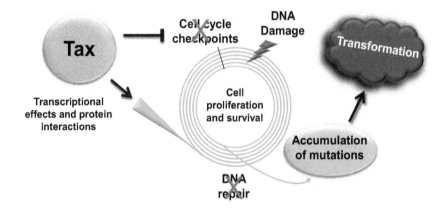

Figure 1. Effects of Tax contribute to cellular transformation: Tax dysregulates cellular gene expression by interacting with cellular proteins and modifying their functions. In the presence of DNA damage (red bolt) Tax interacts with cellular proteins to disrupt cell cycle checkpoints and DNA repair. Persistent activation of NFkB responsive genes such as IL-2, IL-2Rα, and BCL2 drives T cell proliferation and survival. Over many rounds of DNA replication Tax-expressing cells accumulate mutations and promote genome instability, leading to cellular transformation.

6. Conclusions and perspectives

The progression from HTLV-1 infection to the development of ATLL is complicated and not fully understood. The long clinical latency between infection and disease progression makes HTLV-1 an interesting and useful model in which to study multistep oncogenesis [143]. After initial infection, viral proteins including Tax promote viral replication and aid in virus dissemination. HTLV-1 manipulates normal cellular processes to ensure successful replication of the viral genome, which requires entry into and completion of S phase of the cell cycle. Tax inactivates tumor suppressors, interacts with cellular proteins to deregulate cellular gene expression and cell cycle regulation, and inhibits the DDR and apoptosis, all in an effort to disable cell cycle checkpoints and promote cell cycle progression regardless of long-term consequences to the cell (Figure 1). Although the virus remains integrated into the host genome for the life of the host, the virus can successfully replicate and disseminate to other host cells in a matter of days. Thus, accumulation of genetic insults is of little consequence to the virus. Indeed, these insults can be considered an unintended consequence of successful viral replication and dissemination. The ability of Tax to increase the overall cellular mutation rate sets the stage for the development of ATLL. While the effects of Tax on cellular processes are well studied, gaps remain in our understanding of how Tax influences cellular functions due to the interconnectedness of these functions. Advances in animal model systems and experimental systems to study Tax function will help to reveal the complex effects of Tax on interplay between cellular function networks and will increase our ability to identify the key steps involved in HTLV-1 induced leukemogenesis.

Author details

Kendle Pryor[1] and Susan J. Marriott[1,2*]

*Address all correspondence to: susanm@bcm.edu

1 Interdepartmental Program in Cell and Molecular Biology, Baylor College of Medicine, Houston, TX, USA

2 Department of Molecular Virology and Microbiology, Baylor College of Medicine, Houston, TX, USA

References

[1] Proietti, F. A, Carneiro-proietti, A. B, Catalan-soares, B. C, & Murphy, E. L. Global epidemiology of HTLV-I infection and associated diseases. Oncogene (2005). , 24, 6058-6068.

[2] Hinuma, Y, Nagata, K, Hanaoka, M, et al. Adult T-cell leukemia: antigen in an ATL cell line and detection of antibodies to the antigen in human sera. Proc Natl Acad Sci U S A (1981). , 78, 6476-6480.

[3] Yoshida, M, Miyoshi, I, & Hinuma, Y. Isolation and characterization of retrovirus from cell lines of human adult T-cell leukemia and its importance in the disease. Proc Natl Acad Sci USA (1982). , 79, 2031-2035.

[4] Poiesz, B. J, Ruscetti, F. W, Gazdar, A. F, et al. Detection and isolation of type C retrovirus particles from fresh and cultured lymphocytes of a patient with cutaneous T-cell lymphoma. Proc Natl Acad Sci U S A (1980). , 77, 7415-7419.

[5] Gessain, A, Barin, F, Vernant, J. C, et al. Antibodies to human T-lymphotropic virus type I in patients with tropical spastic paraparesis. Lancet (1985). , 2, 407-409.

[6] Osame, M, Usuku, K, Izumo, S, et al. HTLV-I associated myelopathy, a new clinical entity. Lancet (1986). , 1031-1032.

[7] Kajiyama, W, Kashiwagi, S, Ikematsu, H, et al. Intrafamilial transmission of adult T-cell leukemia virus. J Infect Dis (1986). , 154, 851-857.

[8] Kaplan, J. E, Khabbaz, R. F, Murphy, E. L, et al. Male-to-female transmission of human T-cell lymphotropic virus types I and II: association with viral load. The Retrovirus Epidemiology Donor Study Group. J Acquir Immune Defic Syndr Hum Retrovirol (1996). , 12, 193-201.

[9] Murphy, E. L, Figueroa, J. P, Gibbs, W. N, et al. Sexual transmission of human T-lymphotropic virus type I (HTLV-I). Ann Intern Med (1989). , 111, 555-560.

[10] 10 Kannagi, M, Ohashi, T, Harashima, N, et al. Immunological risks of adult T-cell leukemia at primary HTLV-I infection. Trends Microbiol (2004). , 12, 346-352.

[11] Ureta-vidal, A, Angelin-duclos, C, Tortevoye, P, et al. Mother-to-child transmission of human T-cell-leukemia/lymphoma virus type I: implication of high antiviral antibody titer and high proviral load in carrier mothers. Int J Cancer (1999). , 82, 832-836.

[12] Wiktor, S. Z, Pate, E. J, Murphy, E. L, et al. Mother-to-child transmission of human T-cell lymphotropic virus type 1 (HTLV-1) in Jamaica: association with antibodies to envelope glycoprotein (gp46) epitopes. J Acquir Immune Defic Syndr Hum Retrovirol (1993). , 6, 1162-1167.

[13] Shuh, M, & Beilke, M. The human T-cell leukemia virus type 1 (HTLV-1): new insights into the clinical aspects and molecular pathogenesis of adult T-cell leukemia/lympho-ma (ATLL) and tropical spastic paraparesis/HTLV-associated myelopathy (TSP/HAM). Microsc Res Tech (2005). , 68, 176-196.

[14] Yssel, H, De Waal, M. R, et al. Human T cell leukemia/lymphoma virus type I infection of a CD4+ proliferative/cytotoxic T cell clone progresses in at least two distinct phases based on changes in function and phenotype of the infected cells. J Immunol (1989). , 142, 2279-2289.

[15] Akari, H, Ono, F, Sakakibara, I, et al. Simian T cell leukemia virus type I-induced malignant adult T cell leukemia-like disease in a naturally infected African green monkey: implication of CD8+ T cell leukemia. AIDS Res Hum Retroviruses (1998). , 14, 367-371.

[16] Gillet, N, Florins, A, Boxus, M, et al. Mechanisms of leukemogenesis induced by bovine leukemia virus: prospects for novel anti-retroviral therapies in human. Retrovirology (2007).

[17] Mahieux, R, & Gessain, A. HTLV-3/STLV-3 and HTLV-4 viruses: discovery, epidemi-ology, serology and molecular aspects. Viruses (2011). , 3, 1074-1090.

[18] Switzer, W. M, Qari, S. H, Wolfe, N. D, et al. Ancient origin and molecular features of the novel human T-lymphotropic virus type 3 revealed by complete genome analysis. J Virol (2006). , 80, 7427-7438.

[19] Kannian, P, & Green, P. L. Human T Lymphotropic Virus Type 1 (HTLV-1): Molecular Biology and Oncogenesis. Viruses (2010). , 2, 2037-2077.

[20] Franchini, G. Molecular mechanisms of human T-cell leukemia/lymphotropic virus type I infection. Blood (1995). , 86, 3619-3639.

[21] Edwards, D, Fenizia, C, Gold, H, et al. Orf-I and orf-II-encoded proteins in HTLV-1 infection and persistence. Viruses (2011). , 3, 861-885.

[22] Bartoe, J. T, Albrecht, B, Collins, N. D, et al. Functional role of pX open reading frame II of human T-lymphotropic virus type 1 in maintenance of viral loads in vivo. J Virol JID- 0113724 (2000). , 74, 1094-1100.

[23] Collins, N. D, Newbound, G. C, Albrecht, B, et al. Selective ablation of human T-cell lymphotropic virus type 1 reduces viral infectivity in vivo. Blood JID- 7603509 (1998). , 12I.

[24] Robek, M. D, Wong, F. H, & Ratner, L. Human T-cell leukemia virus type 1 pX-I and pX-II open reading frames are dispensable for the immortalization of primary lymphocytes. J Virol (1998). , 72, 4458-4462.

[25] Silverman, L. R, Phipps, A. J, Montgomery, A, et al. Human T-cell lymphotropic virus type 1 open reading frame II-encoded is required for in vivo replication: evidence of in vivo reversion. J Virol (2004). , 30II.

[26] Younis, I, Yamamoto, B, Phipps, A, & Green, P. L. Human T-cell leukemia virus type 1 expressing nonoverlapping tax and rex genes replicates and immortalizes primary human T lymphocytes but fails to replicate and persist in vivo. J Virol (2005). , 79, 14473-14481.

[27] Gatza, M. L, Watt, J. C, & Marriott, S. J. Cellular transformation by the HTLV-I Tax protein, a jack-of-all-trades. Oncogene (2003). , 22, 5141-5149.

[28] Cockerell, G. L, Rovnak, J, Green, P. L, & Chen, I. S. A deletion in the proximal untranslated pX region of human T-cell leukemia virus type II decreases viral replication but not infectivity in vivo. Blood JID- 7603509 (1996). , 87, 1030-1035.

[29] Unge, T, Solomin, L, Mellini, M, et al. The Rex regulatory protein of human T-cell lymphotropic virus type 1 binds specifically to its target site within the viral RNA. Proc Natl Acad Sci USA (1991). , 88, 7145-7149.

[30] Gaudray, G, Gachon, F, Basbous, J, et al. The complementary strand of the human T-cell leukemia virus type 1 RNA genome encodes a bZIP transcription factor that down-regulates viral transcription. J Virol (2002). , 76, 12813-12822.

[31] Arnold, J, Zimmerman, B, Li, M, et al. Human T-cell leukemia virus type-1 antisense-encoded gene, Hbz, promotes T-lymphocyte proliferation. Blood (2008). , 112, 3788-3797.

[32] Grassmann, R, Dengler, C, Muller-fleckenstein, I, et al. Transformation to continuous growth of primary human T lymphocytes by human T cell leukemia virus type I X-region genes transduced by a herpesvirus saimiri vector. Proc Natl Acad Sci USA (1989). , 86, 3551-3355.

[33] Grassmann, R, Berchtold, S, Radant, I, et al. Role of human T-cell leukemia virus type I X region proteins in immortalization of primary human lymphocytes in culture. J Virol (1992). , 66, 4570-4575.

[34] Hinrichs, S. H, Nerenberg, M, Reynolds, R. K, et al. A transgenic mouse model for human neurofibromatosis. Science (1987). , 237, 1340-1343.

[35] Nerenberg, M, Hinrichs, S. H, Reynolds, R. K, et al. The tat gene of human T-lympho-tropic virus type I induces mesenchymal tumors in transgenic mice. Science (1987). , 237, 1324-1329.

[36] Smith, M. R, & Greene, W. C. Type I human T cell leukemia virus Tax protein transforms rat fibroblasts through the cyclic adenosine monophosphate response element binding protein/activating transcription factor pathway. J Clin Invest (1991). , 88, 1038-1042.

[37] Tanaka, A, Takahashi, G, Yamaoka, S, et al. Oncogenic transformation by the tax gene of human T cell leukemia virus type I in vitro. Proc Natl Acad Sci USA (1990). , 87, 1071-1075.

[38] Yamaoka, S, Tobe, T, & Hatanaka, M. Tax protein of human T-cell leukemia virus type I is required for maintenance of the transformed phenotype. Oncogene (1992). , 7, 433-437.

[39] Bruge, J. S, & Erickson, R. L. Identification of a transformation-specific antigen induced by an avian sarcoma virus. Nature (1977). , 269, 346-348.

[40] Paul, R, Schuetze, S, Kozak, S. L, & Kabat, D. A common site for immortalizing proviral integrations in Friend erythroleukemia: molecular cloning and characterization. J Virol (1989). , 63, 4958-4961.

[41] Pozzati, R, Vogel, J, & Jay, G. The human T lymphotropic virus I tax gene can cooperate with the ras oncogene to induce neoplastic transformation of cells. Mol Cell Biol (1990). , 10, 413-417.

[42] Grossman, W. J, Kimata, J. T, Wong, F. H, et al. Development of leukemia in mice transgenic for the tax gene of human T-cell leukemia virus type I. Proc Natl Acad Sci USA (1995). , 92, 1057-1061.

[43] Kitajima, I, Shinohara, T, Bilakovics, J, et al. Ablation of transplanted HTLV-I Tax-transfoprmed tumors in mice by antisense inhibition of NF-kB. Science (1992). , 258, 1792-1795.

[44] Grossman, W. J, & Ratner, L. Cytokine expression and tumorigenicity of large granular lymphocytic leukemia cells from mice transgenic for the tax gene of human T-cell leukemia virus type I. Blood (1997). , 90, 783-794.

[45] Hasegawa, H, Sawa, H, Lewis, M. J, et al. Thymus-derived leukemia-lymphoma in mice transgenic for the Tax gene of human T-lymphotropic virus type I. Nat Med (2006). , 12, 466-472.

[46] Banerjee, P, Tripp, A, Lairmore, M. D, et al. Adult T-cell leukemia/lymphoma development in HTLV-1-infected humanized SCID mice. Blood (2010). , 115, 2640-2648.

[47] Ng PWPIha H, Iwanaga Y, et al. Genome-wide expression changes induced by HTLV-1 Tax: evidence for MLK-3 mixed lineage kinase involvement in Tax-mediated NF-kappa B activation. Oncogene (2001). , 20, 4484-4496.

[48] Pise-masison, C. A, Mahieux, R, Radonovich, M, et al. Human T-lymphotropic virus type I Tax protein utilizes distinct pathways for inhibition that are cell type-dependent. J Biol Chem (2001). , 53.

[49] Semmes, O. J, & Jeang, K-T. Definition of a minimal activation domain in human T-cell leukemia virus type I Tax. J Virol (1995). , 69, 1827-1833.

[50] Smith, M. R, & Greene, W. C. Identification of HTLV-I tax trans-activator mutants exhibiting novel transcriptional phenotypes. Genes Dev (1990). , 4, 1875-1885.

[51] Smith, M. R, & Greene, W. C. Characterization of a novel nuclear localization signal in the HTLV-I tax transactivator protein. Virology (1992). , 187, 316-320.

[52] Adya, N, & Giam, C. Z. Distinct regions in human T-cell lymphotropic virus type I Tax mediate interactions with activator protein CREB and basal transcription factors. J Virol (1995). , 69, 1834-1841.

[53] Ballard, D. W, Bohnlein, E, Lowenthal, J. W, et al. HTLV-1 Tax induces cellular proteins that activate the kB element in the IL-2 receptor gene. Science (1988). , 241, 1652-1655.

[54] Franklin, A. A, Kubik, M. F, Uittenbogaard, M. N, et al. Transactivation by the human T-cell leukemia virus Tax protein is mediated through enhanced binding of ATF-2 and CREB. J Biol Chem (1993). , 268, 21225-21231.

[55] Fujii, M, Niki, T, Mori, T, et al. HTLV-I Tax induces expression of various immediate early serum responsive genes. Oncogene (1991). , 6, 1023-1029.

[56] Fujii, M, Tsuchiya, H, & Seiki, M. HTLV-I Tax has distinct but overlapping domains for transcriptional activation and for enhancer specificity. Oncogene (1991). , 6, 2349-2352.

[57] Fujii, M, Tsuchiya, H, Chuhjo, T, et al. Interaction of HTLV-I Tax1 with causes the aberrant induction of cellular immediate early genes through CArG boxes. Genes Dev (1992). , 67SRF.

[58] Kanno, T, Brown, K, Franzoso, G, & Siebenlist, U. Kinetic analysis of human T-cell leukemia virus type I tax- mediated activation of NF-kappaB. Mol Cell Biol (1994). , 14, 6443-6451.

[59] Low, K. G, Chu, H. M, Tan, Y, et al. Novel interactions between human T-cell leukemia virus type I Tax and activating transcription factor 3 at a cyclic AMP-responsive element. Mol Cell Biol (1994). , 14, 4958-4974.

[60] Ruben, S, Poteat, H, Tan, T, et al. Cellular transcription factors and regulation of IL-2 receptor gene expression by HTLV-I tax gene product. Science (1988). , 241, 89-92.

[61] Winter, H. Y, & Marriott, S. J. Human T-cell leukemia virus type 1 Tax enhances serum response factor DNA binding and alters site selection. J Virol (2007). , 81, 6089-6098.

[62] Yoshida, M. Multiple viral strategies of HTLV-1 for dysregulation of cell growth control. Annu Rev Immunol (2001). , 19, 475-96.

[63] Gonzalez, G. A, & Montminy, M. Cyclic AMP stimulates somatostatin gene transcription by phosphorylation of CREB at serine 133. Cell (1989). , 59, 675-680.

[64] Chrivia, J. C. Kwok RPS, Lamb N, et al. Phosphorylated CREB binds specifically to the nuclear protein CBP. Nature (1993). , 365, 855-859.

[65] Adya, N, Zhao, L. J, Huang, W, et al. Expansion of CREB's DNA recognition specificity by Tax results from interaction with Ala-Ala-Arg at positions 282-284 near the conserved DNA-binding domain of CREB. Proc Natl Acad Sci USA (1994). , 91, 5642-5646.

[66] Kwok RPSLaurance ME, Lundblad JR, et al. Control of cAMP-regulated enhancers by the viral transactivator Tax through CREB and the co-activator CBP. Nature (1996). , 380, 642-646.

[67] Brauweiler, A, Garl, P, Franklin, A. A, et al. A molecular mechanism for human T-cell leukemia virus latency and Tax transactivation. J Biol Chem (1995). , 270, 12814-12822.

[68] Bex, F, Yin, M. J, Burny, A, & Gaynor, R. B. Differential transcriptional activation by human T-cell leukemia virus type 1 Tax mutants is mediated by distinct interactions with CREB binding protein and Mol Cell Biol (1998). , 300.

[69] Bex, F, & Gaynor, R. Regulation of gene expression by HTLV-I Tax protein. Methods: a companion to Methods in Enzymology (1998). , 16, 83-94.

[70] Giebler, H. A, Loring, J. E, Van Orden, K, et al. Anchoring of CREB binding protein to the human T-cell leukemia virus type 1 promoter: A molecular mechanism of tax transactivation. Mol Cell Biol (1997). , 17, 5156-5164.

[71] Harrod, R, Tang, Y, Nicot, C, et al. An exposed KID-like domain in human T-cell lymphotropic virus type 1 Tax is responsible for the recruitment of coactivators CBP/Mol Cell Biol (1998). , 300.

[72] Chen, L. F, & Greene, W. C. Shaping the nuclear action of NF-kappaB. Nat Rev Mol Cell Biol (2004). , 5, 392-401.

[73] Suzuki, T, Hirai, H, Murakami, T, & Yoshida, M. Tax protein of HTLV-1 destabilizes the complexes of NF-kappa B and I kappa B-alpha and induces nuclear translocation of NF-kappa B for transcriptional activation. Oncogene (1995). , 10, 1199-1207.

[74] Chu, Z. L. DiDonato JK, Hawiger J, Ballard DW. The tax oncoprotein of human T-cell leukemia virus type 1 associates with and persistently activates IkappaB kinases containing IKKÃ and IKKÃ¡. J Biol Chem (1998). , 273, 15891-15894.

[75] Chu, Z. L, Shin, Y. A, Yang, J. M, et al. IKKgamma mediates the interaction of cellular IkappaB kinases with the tax transforming protein of human T cell leukemia virus type 1. J Biol Chem (1999). , 274, 15297-15300.

[76] Fu, D. X, Kuo, Y. L, Liu, B. Y, et al. Human T-lymphotropic virus type I Tax activates I-kappa B kinase by inhibiting I-kappa B kinase-associated serine/threonine protein phosphatase 2A. J Biol Chem (2003). , 278, 1487-1493.

[77] Brockman, J. A, Scherer, D. C, Mckinsey, T. A, et al. Coupling of a signal response domain in I kappa B alpha to multiple pathways for NF-kappa B activation. Mol Cell Biol (1995). , 15, 2809-2818.

[78] Watanabe, M, Muramatsu, M, Hirai, H, et al. HTLV-I encoded Tax in association with NF-kappaB precursor enhances nuclear localization of NF-kappaB p50 and p65 in transfected cells. Oncogene (1993). , 105.

[79] Lacoste, J, Cohen, L, & Hiscott, J. NF-kappa B activity in T cells stably expressing the Tax protein of human T cell lymphotropic virus type I. Virology (1991). , 184, 553-562.

[80] Robek, M. D, & Ratner, L. Immortalization of CD4 + and CD8 + T lymphocytes by human T- cell leukemia virus type 1 Tax mutants expressed in a functional molecular clone. J Virol (1999). , 73, 4856-4865.

[81] Rosin, O, Koch, C, Schmitt, I, et al. A human T-cell leukemia virus Tax variant incapable of activating NF- K B retains its immortalizing potential for primary T-lymphocytes. J Biol Chem (1998). , 273, 6698-6703.

[82] Yamaoka, S, Inoue, H, Sakurai, M, et al. Constitutive activation of NF-kB is essential for transformation of rat fibroblasts by the human T-cell leukemia virus type I Tax protein. EMBO J (1996). , 15, 873-887.

[83] Lemoine, F. J, Kao, S. Y, & Marriott, S. J. Suppression of DNA Repair by HTLV-I Tax correlates with Tax transactivation of PCNA gene expression. AIDS Res Hum Retro-viruses (2000). , 16, 1623-1627.

[84] Miyake, H, Suzuki, T, Hirai, H, & Yoshida, M. Trans-activator Tax of human T-cell leukemia virus type 1 enhances mutation frequency of the cellular genome. Virology (1999). , 253, 155-161.

[85] Sancar, A, Lindsey-boltz, L. A, Unsal-kaccmaz, K, & Linn, S. MOLECULAR MECHA-NISMS OF MAMMALIAN DNA REPAIR AND THE DNA DAMAGE CHECK-POINTS. Annu Rev Biochem (2004). , 73, 39-85.

[86] Sobol, R. W, Horton, J. K, Kuhn, R, et al. Requirement of mammalian DNA polymerase-beta in base-excision repair. Nature (1996). , 379, 183-186.

[87] Wood, R. D, & Shivji, M. K. Which DNA polymerases are used for DNA-repair in eukaryotes? Carcinogenesis (1997). , 18, 605-610.

[88] Philpott, S. M, & Buehring, G. C. Defective DNA repair in cells with human T-cell leukemia bovine leukemia viruses: Role of tax gene. J Natl Cancer Inst (1999). , 91, 933-942.

[89] Jeang, K. T, Widen, S. G, Semmes, O. J, & Wilson, S. H. HTLV-I trans-activator protein, Tax, is a trans-repressor of the human β-polymerase gene. Science (1990). , 247, 1082-1084.

[90] Gary, R, Kim, K, Cornelius, H. L, et al. Proliferating cell nuclear antigen facilitates excision in long- patch base excision repair. J Biol Chem (1999). , 274, 4354-4363.

[91] Matsumoto, Y, & Kim, K. Excision of deoxyribose phosphate residues by DNA polymerase beta during DNA repair. Science (1995). , 269, 699-702.

[92] Li, R, Waga, S, Hannon, G. J, et al. Differential effects by the CDK inhibitor on PCNA-dependent DNA replication and repair. Nature (1994). , 21.

[93] Ressler, S, Morris, G. F, & Marriott, S. J. Human T-cell leukemia virus type 1 Tax transactivates the human proliferating cell nuclear antigen promoter. J Virol (1997). , 71, 1181-1190.

[94] Kao, S. Y, & Marriott, S. J. Disruption of nucleotide excision repair by the human T-cell leukemia virus type 1 Tax protein. J Virol (1999). , 73, 4299-4304.

[95] Lemoine, F. J, Kao, S. Y, & Marriott, S. J. Suppression of DNA Repair by HTLV-I Tax correlates with Tax transactivation of PCNA gene expression. AIDS Res Hum Retroviruses (2000). , 16, 1623-1627.

[96] Driscoll, O, & Jeggo, M. PA. The role of double-strand break repair- insights from human genetics. Nat Rev Genet (2006). , 7, 45-54.

[97] Ducu, R. I, Dayaram, T, & Marriott, S. J. The HTLV-1 Tax oncoprotein represses Ku80 gene expression. Virology (2011). , 416, 1-8.

[98] Majone, F, Luisetto, R, Zamboni, D, et al. Ku protein as a potential human T-cell leukemia virus type 1 (HTLV-1) Tax target in clastogenic chromosomal instability of mammalian cells. Retrovirology (2005).

[99] Chandhasin, C, Ducu, R. I, Berkovich, E, et al. Human T-cell leukemia virus type 1 tax attenuates the ATM-mediated cellular DNA damage response. J Virol (2008). , 82, 6952-6961.

[100] Majone, F, & Jeang, K. T. Clastogenic effect of the human T-cell leukemia virus type I tax oncoprotein correlates with unstabilized DNA breaks. J Biol Chem (2000). , 275, 32906-32910.

[101] Majone, F, Semmes, O. J, & Jeang, K-T. Induction of micronuclei by HTLV-I Tax: a cellular assay for function. Virology (1993). , 193, 456-459.

[102] Sherr, C. J. G. phase progression: cycling on cue. Cell (1994). , 79, 551-555.

[103] Lemasson, I, Thebault, S, Sardet, C, et al. Activation of E2F-mediated transcription by human T-cell leukemia virus type I Tax protein in a INK4A)-negative T-cell line. J Biol Chem (1998). , 16.

[104] Haller, K, Wu, Y, Derow, E, et al. Physical interaction of human T-cell leukemia virus type 1 tax with cyclin-dependent kinase 4 stimulates the phosphorylation of retinoblastoma protein. Mol Cell Biol (2002). , 22, 3327-3338.

[105] Ohtani, K, Iwanaga, R, Arai, M, et al. Cell type-specific E2F activation and cell cycle progression induced by the oncogene product Tax of human T-cell leukemia virus type I. J Biol Chem JID- 2985121R (2000). , 275, 11154-11163.

[106] Lemasson, I. Thâ€šbault S, Sardet C, et al. Activation of E2F-mediated transcription by human T-cell leukemia virus type I tax protein in a INK4A-negative T-cell line. J Biol Chem (1998). , 16.

[107] Levine, A. J. p. the cellular gatekeeper for growth and division. Cell (1997). , 88, 323-331.

[108] Akagi, T, Ono, H, & Shimotohno, K. Expression of cell-cycle regulatory genes in HTLV-I infected T- cell lines: Possible involvement of Tax1 in the altered expression of cyclin D2, Ink4 and p21 Waf1/Cip1/Sdi1. Oncogene (1996). , 18.

[109] Kawata, S, Ariumi, Y, & Shimotohno, K. p. Waf1/Cip1/Sdi1) prevents apoptosis as well as stimulates growth in cells transformed or immortalized by human T-cell leukemia virus type 1-encoded tax. J Virol (2003). , 77, 7291-7299.

[110] Lemoine, F. J, Marriott, S. J, & Accelerated, G. phase progression induced by the human T cell leukemia virus type I (HTLV-I) Tax oncoprotein. J Biol Chem (2001). , 276, 31851-31857.

[111] Cereseto, A, Diella, F, Mulloy, J. C, et al. functional impairment and high p21waf1/cip1 expression in human T-cell lymphotropic/leukemia virus type I-transformed T cells. Blood (1996). , 53.

[112] Hatta, Y, & Koeffler, H. P. Role of tumor suppressor genes in the development of adult T cell leukemia/lymphoma (ATLL). Leukemia (2002). , 16, 1069-1085.

[113] Ariumi, Y, Yamaoka, S, Lin, J. Y, et al. HTLV-1 tax oncoprotein represses the trans-activation function through coactivator CBP sequestration. Oncogene (2000). , 53.

[114] Suzuki, T, Uchida-toita, M, & Yoshida, M. Tax protein of HTLV-1 inhibits CBP/transcription by interfering with recruitment of CBP/p300 onto DNA element of E-box or p53 binding site. Oncogene (1999). , 300.

[115] Van Orden, K, Giebler, H. A, Lemasson, I, et al. Binding of to the KIX domain of CREB binding protein. A potential link to human T-cell leukemia virus type I-associated leukemogenesis. J Biol Chem (1999). , 53.

[116] Pise-masison, C. A, Radonovich, M, Sakaguchi, K, et al. Phosphorylation of a novel pathway for p53 inactivation in human T-cell lymphotropic virus type 1-transformed cells. J Virol (1998). , 53.

[117] Pise-masison, C. A, Mahieux, R, Jiang, H, et al. Inactivation of by human T-cell lymphotropic virus type 1 Tax requires activation of the NF-kB pathway and is dependent on p53 phosphorylation. Mol Cell Biol (2000). , 53.

[118] Jeong, S. J, Radonovich, M, & Brady, J. N. Pise Masison CA. HTLV-I Tax induces a novel interaction between RelA and p53 which results in inhibition of p53 transcriptional activity. Blood (2004). , 65.

[119] Peter, M, & Herskowitz, I. Joining the complex: cyclin-dependent kinase inhibitory proteins and the cell cycle. Cell (1994). , 79, 181-184.

[120] Sherr, C, & Roberts, J. M. Inhibitors of mammalian G1 cyclin-dependent kinases. Genes Dev (1995). , 9, 1149-1163.

[121] Hannon, G. J, & Beach, D. p. INK4B is a potential effector of TGF-beta-induced cell cycle arrest. Nature JID- 0410462 (1994). , 371, 257-261.

[122] Low, K. G, Dorner, L. F, Fernando, D. B, et al. Human T-cell leukemia virus type 1 tax releases cell cycle arrest induced by INK4a. J Virol (1997). , 16.

[123] Suzuki, T, Kitao, S, Matsushime, H, & Yoshida, M. HTLV-1 Tax protein interacts with cyclin-dependent kinase inhibitor and counteracts its inhibitory activity towards CDK4. EMBO J (1996). , 16INK4A.

[124] Iwanaga, R, Ohtani, K, Hayashi, T, & Nakamura, M. Molecular mechanism of cell cycle progression induced by the oncogene product Tax of human T-cell leukemia virus type I. Oncogene (2001). , 20, 2055-2067.

[125] Suzuki, T, Narita, T, Uchida-toita, M, & Yoshida, M. Down-regulation of the INK4 family of cyclin-dependent kinase inhibitors by tax protein of HTLV-1 through two distinct mechanisms. Virology (1999). , 259, 384-391.

[126] Kibler, K. V, & Jeang, K. T. CREB/ATF-dependent repression of cyclin a by human T-cell leukemia virus type 1 Tax protein. J Virol (2001). , 75, 2161-2173.

[127] Chieco-bianchi, L, & Saggioro, D. DelMistro A, et al. Chromosome damage induced in cord blood T-lymphocytes infected in vitro by HTLV-I. Leukemia (1988). s-232s.

[128] Fujimoto, T, Hatta, T, Itoyama, T, et al. High rate of chromosomal abnormalities in HTLV-I-infected T-cell colonies derived from prodromal phase of adult T-cell leukemia: A study of IL-2-stimulated colony formation in methylcellulose. Cancer Genet Cytogenet (1999). , 109, 1-13.

[129] Itoyama, T, Sadamori, N, Tokunaga, S, et al. Cytogenetic studies of human T-cell leukemia virus type I carriers. A family study. Cancer Genet Cytogenet (1990). , 49, 157-163.

[130] Kamada, N, Sakurai, M, Miyamoto, K, et al. Chromosome abnormalities in adult T-cell leukemia/lymphoma: a karyotype review committee report. Cancer Res (1992). , 52, 1482-1493.

[131] Maruyama, K, Fukushima, T, Kawamura, K, & Mochizuki, S. Chromosome and gene rearrangements in immortalized human lymphocytes infected with human T-lymphotropic virus type I. Cancer Res (1990). s-5702s.

[132] Miyamoto, K, Tomita, N, Ishii, A, et al. Chromosome abnormalities of leukemia cells in adult aptients with T-cell leukemia. J Natl Can Instit (1984). , 73, 353-362.

[133] Rowley, J. D, Haren, J. M, Wong-staal, F, Franchini, G, Gallo, R. C, Blattner, W, et al. Chromosome patterns in cells from patients positive for human T-cell leukemia/lymphoma virus. Human T-cell leukemia/lymphoma virus. New York: Cold Spring Harbor Laboratory, (1984). , 1984, 85-89.

[134] Sadamori, N. Cytogenetic implication in adult T-cell leukemia. A hypothesis of leukemogenesis. Cancer Genet Cytogenet (1991). , 51, 131-136.

[135] Whang-peng, J. Chen YMA, Knutsen T, et al. Chromosome studies in HTLV-I,-II, and HTLV-1,-2 cell lines infected in vivo and in vitro. J Acquir Immune Defic Syndr Hum Retrovirol (1993). , 6, 930-940.

[136] Park, H. U, Jeong, J. H, Chung, J. H, & Brady, J. N. Human T-cell leukemia virus type 1 Tax interacts with Chk1 and attenuates DNA-damage induced G2 arrest mediated by Chk1. Oncogene (2004). , 23, 4966-4974.

[137] Gupta, S. K, Guo, X, Durkin, S. S, et al. Human T-cell leukemia virus type 1 tax oncoprotein prevents DNA damage-induced chromatin egress of hyperphosphorylated Chk2. J Biol Chem (2007). , 282, 29431-29440.

[138] Lavia, P, Mileo, A. M, Giordano, A, & Paggi, M. G. Emerging roles of DNA tumor viruses in cell proliferation: new insights into genomic instability. Oncogene (2003). , 22, 6508-6516.

[139] Parry, J. M, & Parry, E. M. Comparison of tests for aneuploidy. Mutation Research (1987). , 181, 267-287.

[140] Thompson, E. J, & Perry, P. E. The identification of micronucleated chromosomes: a possible assay for aneuploidy. Mutagenesis (1988). , 3, 415-418.

[141] Jin, D. Y, Spencer, F, & Jeang, K. T. Human T cell leukemia virus type 1 oncoprotein tax targets the human mitotic checkpoint protein MAD1. Cell (1998). , 93, 81-91.

[142] Liu, B, Liang, M. H, Kuo, Y. L, et al. Human T-lymphotropic virus type 1 oncoprotein tax promotes unscheduled degradation of Pds1p/securin and Clb2p/cyclin B1 and causes chromosomal instability. Mol Cell Biol (2003). , 23, 5269-5281.

[143] Yasunaga, J, & Matsuoka, M. Human T-cell leukemia virus type I induces adult T-cell leukemia: from clinical aspects to molecular mechanisms. Cancer Control (2007). , 14, 133-140.

Chapter 4

Glycan Profiling of Adult T-Cell Leukemia (ATL) Cells with the High Resolution Lectin Microarrays

Hidekatsu Iha and Masao Yamada

Additional information is available at the end of the chapter

1. Introduction

1.1. Roles of glycans on diverse aspects of biological activities

Regardless of species, all the living organisms have poly-saccharides called glycans in their cellular surfaces or even inside the cells. The biological roles of carbohydrates are particularly important in the assembly of complex multicellular organs, which requires interactions between cells and the surrounding matrix. All cells and numerous macromolecules in nature carry an array of covalently attached sugars (monosaccharides) or sugar chains (oligosaccharides). Because many glycans are on the outer surface of cells or secreted macromolecules, they are acting to modulate or mediate a wide variety of events in cell to cell, cell with matrix, and cell with proteins or lipids critical to the development and function of complex forms of multicellular organisms (Rademacheret al., 1988; Sharon and Lis, 1993; Varki, 1993).

Glycans also function as mediators in the interactions between different organisms, for example, between hosts and infectious agents or symbionts. In addition, simple, rapidly turning over, protein-bound glycans are abundant within the nucleus and cytoplasm, where they act as regulatory switches. Therefore, as a complete paradigm of biology, glycans should be included quite often in covalent combination with other macromolecules such as glycoproteins and glycolipids, so called glycoconjugates (Gagneux and Varki, 1999).

Figure 1 provides a listing of known glycan-protein or glycan-lipid linkages in nature. The common classes of glycans found in or on eukaryotic cells are primarily defined according to the nature of the linkage to the targets. A glycoprotein is a glycoconjugate in which a protein carries one or more glycans covalently attached to a polypeptide backbone, usually via N or O linkages. An N-glycan (N or asparagine-linked oligosaccharide) is a sugar chain covalently attached to an asparagine residue of a polypeptide chain at the consensus peptide sequence:

Asn-X-Ser/Thr. A mucin is a large glycoprotein that carries many O-glycans that are clustered. A proteoglycan is a glycoconjugate that has one or more glycosaminoglycan (GAG) chains attached to a "core protein" through a typical core region ending in a xylose residue that is linked to the hydroxyl group of a serine residue. The distinction between a proteoglycan and a glycoprotein is otherwise arbitrary, because some proteoglycan polypeptides carry both glycosaminoglycan chains and different O- and N-glycans. A glycophosphatidylinositol anchor is a glycan bridge between phosphatidylinositol and a phosphoethanolamine that is in amide linkage to the carboxyl terminus of a protein. This structure typically constitutes the only anchor to the lipid bilayer membrane for such proteins. A glycosphingolipid (often called a glycolipid) consists of a glycan usually attached via glucose or galactose to the terminal primary hydroxyl group of the lipid moiety ceramide, which is composed of a long chain base (sphingosine) and a fatty acid. Glycolipids can be neutral or anionic. A ganglioside is an anionic glycolipid containing one or more residues of sialic acid. It should be noted that these represent only the most common classes of glycans reported in eukaryotic cells. There are several other less common types found on one or the other side of the cell membrane in animal cells (Varki, 1997; Fuster and Esko, 2005).

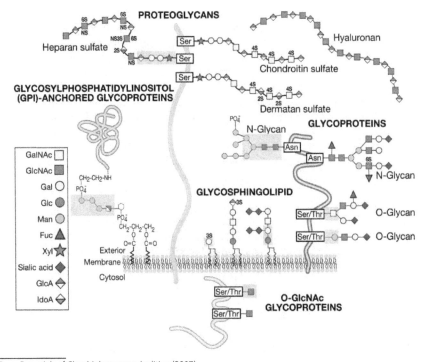

From Essentials of Glycobiology second edition (2007)

Figure 1. Glycans on surface or inside the cells

As can be imagined from their ubiquitous and complex nature, the biological roles of glycans are quite diverse spanning the spectrum from those that are subtle to those that are crucial for the development, growth, function, or survival of an organism. The diverse functions attributed to glycans can be divided into two general categories: (i) structural and modulatory functions (involving the glycans themselves or their modulation of the molecules to which they are attached) and (ii) specific recognition of glycans by glycan-binding proteins, called lectin. Expression of certain sets of glycans in intact organisms are found exquisitely specific temporal and spatial patterns those glycans in relation to cellular activation, embryonic development, organogenesis, and differentiation. Certain relatively specific changes in expression of glycans are also often found in the course of transformation and progression to malignancy, as well as other pathological situations such as inflammation. These spatially and temporally controlled patterns of glycan expression imply the involvement of glycans in many normal and pathological processes, the precise mechanisms of which are not well understood (Theocharis, 2010; Hynes and Naba, 2012).

2. Glycans as the markers of cancer

Tumor cells undergo alteration of intracellular signalings to promote cell cycle progression and rapid growth, adhere to a variety of other cell types and cell matrices, and invade tissues. Embryonic development and cellular activation in vertebrates are typically accompanied by changes in cellular glycosylation profiles. It is therefore rational that glycosylation changes are also a typical feature of malignant transformation and tumor progression. The earliest evidence came from observing that plant lectins showed enhanced binding to and agglutination of tumor cells. Next, it was found that in vitro transformation was frequently accompanied by a general increase in the size of metabolically labeled glycopeptides produced by trypsinization of surface molecules from cancer cells (Hakomori and Kannagi, 1983). With the advent of monoclonal antibody technology in the late 1970s, investigators found many "tumor-specific" antibodies which were directed against glycan epitopes, especially those borne on glycosphingolipids (Feizi, 1985). In most cases, further studies showed that these epitopes were also expressed in embryonic tissues and, in a few cell types, in the normal adult (Fukuda, 1996). Significant correlations between certain types of altered glycosylation and the prognosis of tumor-bearing animals or patients increased interest in these changes. In several instances, in vitro cellular assays and in vivo animal studies have further supported the view that these changes are critical to aspects of tumor cell behavior (Kannagi et al., 2004).

3. HTLV-1 causes complicated forms of diseases to human

Human T-lymphotropic virus type 1 (HTLV-1) is the first and unique oncogenic retrovirus that infects 20 million more people worldwide (Hinuma et al., 1992; Proietti et al., 2005; Gonçalves et al., 2010; Sonoda et al., 2011). Among these infected individuals, 2 to 5% develop aggressive and mostly fetal adult T cell leukemia/lymphoma: ATL (Yoshida, 2010; Iwanaga et al., 2010), and a further 1 to 2% develop a variety of chronic inflammatory syndromes, known as HTLV-1–associated myelopathy/tropical spastic paraparesis: HAM/TSP (Osame et al., 1986) and HTLV-1–associated uveitis: HU (Mochizuki et al., 1992). HTLV-1 has also linked, even with less definitive epidemiologic proof, dermatitis (La Grenade et al., 1990; Amano et al., 2011), polymyositis (Inose et al., 1992), synovitis (Nishioka et al., 1989; Sowa, 1992), thyroiditis (Kawai et al., 1991) and bronchio-alveolar pneumonitis (Kimura et al., 1989). While the pathophysiologies of patients with HAM/TSP and HU have relatively been well controlled, the efficacy of present treatment procedures to ATL are quite insufficient and leading ATL as one of the worst blood cell malignancies to cure (Olière et al., 2011; Tsukasaki, 2012). Researchers hence are trying to develop any diagnostic tools enabling to identify the high risk carriers (who may develop ATL) in the early phase of infection.

HTLV-1 seropositivity is corresponding to the modes of transmission: from mother to child, predominantly through breast feeding as the initiation for common course of ATL development (Hino et al., 1985); via sexual intercourse and via parenteral transmission by transfusion of infected cellular blood products or sharing of needles and syringes as the courses for HAM/TSP or HU onset (Manns et al., 1991, Proyetti 2005). HTLV-1 infection mostly happens to CD4 T-lymphocytes (Gallo et al., 1982), and multiple viral proteins are produced from the provirus. Among those viral proteins, HTLV-1 trans-activator protein Tax, which promotes the early events of oncogenic process including its own long-terminal-repeat (LTR) transcription (Fujisawa et al., 1985), activates several major cellular transcription factor pathways, such as nuclear factor (NF)-kappaB (Ruben et al., 1988; Yamaoka et al., 1998), cAMP response element binding protein (CREB)/AP-1 transcription factor (ATF, Andrisani et al., 1990; Xu et al., 1990; Himes, 1993), and serum response factor (SRF, Fujii et al., 1991), all of which eventually mediate viral immortalization. Tax targeted genes include interleukin (IL)-2 and the IL-2alpha receptor (Tac or CD25), which initiate and sustain an autocrine pathway of T-cell activation (Ruben et al., 1988). On the late stage of ATL development, infected cell undergoes extensive genetic alterations and some of these populations induce aberrant micro-RNA expression (Yeung et al., 2008) resulting in overexpression of NIK, a strongest NF-kappaB inducing MAP3 kinase, and cells eventually become independent from Tax-mediated NF-kappaB signaling (Yamagishi et al., 2012). Finally, another HTLV-1 encoded oncogenic trans-activator, HTLV-1-basic-zipper protein (HBZ), induces Foxp3, a transcription factor necessary for maintenance of the regulatory T-cell phenotype, to develop immune-suppressive environment which is favorable to establish malignant phenotype of ATL (Gaudray et al., 2002; Satou et al., 2008).

ATL cells display several characteristic 'ATL-specific' cell surface markers such as CD25, OX40, and TSLC1 (Teshigawara et al., 1985; Baum et al., 1994; Sasaki et al., 2005). Japanese HTLV-1 cohort study group, however, have reported that the most reliable molecular based definitive risk factors for the development of ATL among asymptomatic HTLV-1 carriers are baseline proviral load higher than 4 copies/100 peripheral blood mononuclear cells. Although advanced age, family history of ATL, and first opportunity for HTLV-1 testing during treatment for other diseases have also determined as the independent risk factors for ATL prognosis (Iwanaga et al., 2010), we still do not know how many cellular factors and to what extent in HTLV-1 infected subjects contribute to ATL pathogenesis nor which biomarkers distinctly determine the wide ranges of ATL pathological conditions (i.e., smoldering, chronic or acute leukemia or lymphoma).

4. Linkage between efficacy and subtypes of ATL symptoms

Shimoyama (1991) first proposed the diagnostic criteria to classify four clinical subtypes of ATL: (1) Smoldering type, 5% or more abnormal lymphocytes of T-cell nature in PBL, no hypercalcaemia (corrected calcium level less than 2.74 mmol/l), lactate dehydrogenase (LDH) value of up to 1.5 x the normal upper limit, no lymphadenopathy, no involvement of liver, spleen, central nervous system (CNS), bone and gastrointestinal tract, and neither ascites nor pleural effusion. Skin and pulmonary lesion(s) may be present. (2) Chronic type, absolute lymphocytosis (4×10^9/l or more) with T-lymphocytosis more than 3.5×10^9/l, LDH value up to twice the normal upper limit, no hypercalcaemia, no involvement of CNS, bone and gastrointestinal tract, and neither ascites nor pleural effusion. Lymphadenopathy and involvement of liver, spleen, skin, and lung may be present, and 5% or more abnormal T-lymphocytes are seen in PBL in most cases. (3) Lymphoma type, no lymphocytosis, 1% or less abnormal T-lymphocytes, and histologically-proven lymphadenopathy with or without extranodal lesions. (4) Acute type, remaining ATL patients who have usually leukemic manifestation and tumor lesions, but are not classified as any of the three other types. Smoldering and chronic subtypes are indolent but once these group become acute subtype, the mean survival period even with the best protocol of chemotherapy, mLSG15, is only 13 months and overall two year survival ratio is only 25% (Tsukasaki, 2012).

To improve the poor prognosis of ATL, new chemical combinations or new biological treatment, including antibody targeting, immune activation by vaccination or bone marrow transplantation have developed (Tsukasaki et al., 2009; Nasr et al., 2011; Nakano and Watanabe, 2012).

Bazarbachi and his colleagues reported that treatment in combination of anti-virus drug zidovudine (AZT) and interferon-alpha (IFN-α) have dramatically improved the five year survival rate of ATL patients up to 46% (Bazarbachi et al., 2010). AZT/ IFN-α protocol is the most promising for ATL treatment at present but it is not omnipotent for the following reason. This study was applied for all four different ATL subtypes and achieved 77% five-year survival rate for smoldering/chronic and 28% for acute subtype respectively. For lymphoma subtype however this protocol had no effects with 7-month median and no further survival beyond 18 month after treatment. This result clearly indicated that the novel fine and reliable subtype-specific diagnostics for asymptomatic but high-risk carriers are urgently required.

5. Glycans as the potential biomarkers for ATL subtypes

It's been thirty seven years since Van Beek reported the relationship between the malignancy and glycoprotein distribution on the surface of leukemic cells (Van Beek et al., 1975). Then

Dnistrian claimed the plasma lipid-bound sialic acid as a diagnostic marker for hematologic tumors as well as other carcinomas (Dnistrian and Schwartz, 1981). Ohmori and his colleagues first reported that a distinct type of sialyl Lewis X antigen is selectively expressed on helper memory T cells and also on ATL cells which are defined by the monoclonal antibody 2F3 (Ohmori et al., 1993) and Sanada et al. reported that ATL patient's levels of serum hyaluronic acid moved in parallel with the clinical activity of their disease (Sanada et al., 1999). These reports clearly indicate that glycans should play very important roles on a tumorigenic development of hematologic malignancy. However the complicated nature of carbohydrates have hindered the development of diagnostic tools providing a statistically reliable values which eventually define the linkage between glycans and tumor malignancies. To do so, this device should quantitate the amount of multiple forms of glycans at one time and perform multivariate analysis.

6. Lectin microarray as the profiler of ATL cell pathogenic development

There are basically three major processes in glycomics research: (1) glycan synthesis, (2) glycan structural analysis and (3) glycan functional analysis. Glycan structural analysis is considered the first priority as it elucidates the biological functions of the glycans. It is not that simple as DNA or peptide sequencing is resolving most of questions because glycans are not linear-chain molecules but having varieties of branching molecular structures.

Our strategy in glycomics takes a different approach from that used in genomics. We have adopted the use of lectins as so-called "biological decipherers" of glycan structures, capitalizing on their binding specificity to glycan structures. Further, a microarray strategy allows us to utilize a number of lectins with different specificity thereby enabling 'glycome' analyses of small sample amounts with high sensitivity and high throughput (Kuno A et al., 2005).

Mass spectroscopy (MS) is one possible alternative approach used in glycomic structural analysis. MS potentially is a very powerful tool; however it is not versatile enough to be used since MS is not suitable for differentiation of isomers, analysis of O-glycans, and not applicable for crude samples. MS basically requires fairly large samples sizes (>100 μg of proteins) due to its low resolution. Additionally, pre-treatment of the samples on glycan structural analysis by MS is time consuming and bothersome (Pre-treatments requires the isolation of glycoproteins, cleaving of the glycans from the core proteins, and those labeling). From those practical views, the lectin microarray methodology is potentially very powerful for glycomic analysis: (1) quick and easy to use: structural profiling can be performed directly on fluorescence-labeled glycoproteins; no need of glycan cleavage from proteins, (2) highly sensitive: 1 - 100 ng order of glycoproteins is good enough, and (3) high-throughput: benefit of microarray format. To note however, the inference performance of the lectin microarray may not be sufficient as that of MS.

One of the most noteworthy features of basic glycomics research is the weak interaction of glycans and lectins (by more than two orders of magnitude) compared with that of antibodies and antigens as well as nucleotide's hydrogen bonds. This fact inevitably created a need for a new technology which is capable of detecting very weak glycan-lectin interactions directly from a liquid phase without any washing process that is indispensable in DNA microarrays or in ELISA assays to remove non-specific bindings and extra amounts of labeled molecules floating in the liquid phase.

The GlycoStation™ and LecChip™ (lectin microarray containing 45 different lectins immobilized on a slide glass, GP Biosciences, Japan) employs novel 'evanescent-field fluorescence excitation (EFFEX)' technologies were thus developed to obtain specific and highly sensitive glycan-lectin interactions without washing (Fig. 2A). In this scanner, the excitation light bundle incidents into a slide glass from the edge at an appropriate incident angle to form total internal reflection at the interfaces between slide glass and sample solution. A configuration adopted in this scanner will be the simplest and easiest one which is able to generate the evanescent-filed as large as slide glass size (US Patent 6,787,364,2004). Under such conditions, an evanescent-field is formed on the surface of the lower refractive index side. The strength of evanescent-field decreases exponentially as the distance increases from the slide surface. The evanescent-field depth defined by the distance that the field strength drops to $1/e$ ranges from 100 nm to 200nm (it depends on the wavelength of excitation light adopted). Because of this nature, floating glycans in a liquid phase only shows very low excitation in the evanescent field, but glycans interacting with lectins can be excited effectively (Fig. 2B) and very weak molecular interactions between glycans and lectins are monitored efficiently from the liquid phase samples without any washing (Fig. 2C). GlycoStation can be used for screening and understanding how partial glycan structures on cell surfaces change depending on the condition of the cells (i.e., cancer, disease, cell differentiation stage and so on); and to elucidate the roles glycans play and to understand the correlation between glycoforms and cell conditions. We therefore applied this system for evaluation of ATL cell pathogenic developments.

7. Lectin microarray reveals ATL cell specific lectin binding profiles

Conventional diagnosis on leukemia/lymphoma basically takes the following three methods, (1) microscopic observation of tumor cell morphologies with staining by Giemsa, HE/MPO, (2) quantitation of cellular surface marker molecules (glycoproteins usually) with fluorescence activated cell sorter (FACS), and (3) karyotypic or molecular genetic diagnosis on chromosome DNA. All these techniques require expertise and sometimes, especially through microscopic observations, diagnosis varies because of their less quantitative nature.

In the case of ATL diagnosis, as mentioned above, four different subtypes are classified by PBL counts and antibodies against HTLV-1 glycoproteins, biochemical values (calcium and LDH), and morphological observations of HTLV-1 infected lymphocytes. Cellular surface markers such as CD4, CD25 and provirus load are also measured for detailed analysis. Even with these criteria, however, early diagnosis for these subtype classification is not applicable.

Therefore, we may explore to see how accurately lectin microarray identifies the subtypes of ATL with multiple lectin-glycan interaction (LGI) values by Lectin array/ Glycostation. As a preliminary experiment, we evaluated the LGI values of the following six different of

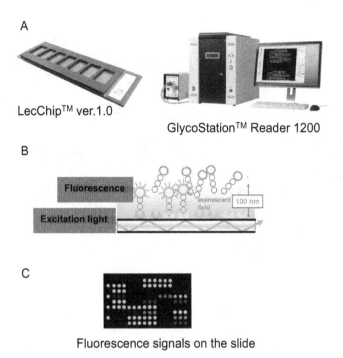

A

LecChip™ ver.1.0

GlycoStation™ Reader 1200

B

Fluorescence

evanescent field | 100 nm

Excitation light

C

Fluorescence signals on the slide

Figure 2. Principles and devices of LecChip lectin microarray

cell, (1) two subjects of CD3+, CD4+ Helper T-cells (PBL-M, PBL-I) from healthy volunteers, (2) two subjects of HTLV-1 transformed cells (C8166, ED), and (3) two subjects of CD25+ ATL patient's peripheral blood cells (ATL4, ATL9). While PBL showed uniformly distributed relatively small cells, all ATL cells are large (twice as PBL-M or -I). ATL cells show aggregation clusters (glycans might be involved in these morphogenesis) and the extents of aggregation in these four subjects are, from high to low, in order of C8166, ATL4, ATL9 and ED (no aggregation, Fig. 3A). Then, we evaluated NF-κB activation level of these six subjects by western blot (WB) analysis (Fig. 3B). To evaluate how NF-κB is activated, cellular lysates from six subjects were fractionated into cytoplasmic (Cyt) and nuclear (Nuc) fractions. PBLs from healthy carriers, of course, don't express Tax (lane 1 to 4), C8166 expresses Tax in highest level (lane 8, 9), ATL4 and AT9 express less amount (lane 5 to 8) and ED doesn't (lane 11, 12). In accordance with Tax expression, the amount of I-κBα was decreased in C8166 most and in ATL4 next. Two PBLs show the same levels of I-κBα and in the case of ATL9 and ED, I-κBα was accumulated in cytoplasm with very high amount. p65, a main species of NF-κB then accumulated in nucleus in C8166 most and, surprisingly, ATL9 and ED also showed its accumulation with almost equivalent amount of ATL4.

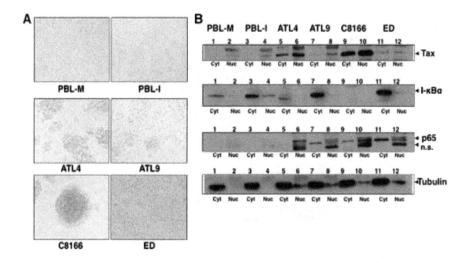

Figure 3. Cell aggregation characteristics and Tax-NF-κB activation properties of ATL cells

From these observations, we concluded the characterizations of these cells as follows; (1) C8166 and ATL4 are to be characterized as Tax-high and heavy cell aggregation types, (2) ATL9 is Tax-low and moderate cell aggregation type, and (3) ED is no-Tax and dispersed type. One can imagine that the former type is sticky and accumulate easily to peripheral lymph nodes and the latter is circulating in the blood vessels as leukemic cells.

Taking cytological characteristics mentioned above into consideration, we evaluated membrane glycoprotein fractions extracted from the six subjects by LecChip™ / GlycoStation™. Two PBLs showed very similar glycan profiles, but the other ATL samples showed various glycan profiles. Concretely speaking, the expression levels of glycans interacting with nine different lectins (AAL, MAL, PHA(E), DSA, ACG, LEL, Jacalin, ACA, WGA) were higher in C8166 comparing with PBL, and inversely seven different lectins (SNA, SSA, TJA-I, NPA, GNA, HHL Calsepa) showed lower interaction to those of C8166. In the case of ATL4, eight out of nine lectins (except for WGA) listed in C8166 showed higher interactions, and the same set of seven lectins showed lower profiles. One thing we have to emphasize here for ATL4 is that SNA, SSA, TJA-I which have binding specificity to α 2,3-NeuAc showed significantly lower expression comparing with others. In the case of ATL9, the six lectin interactions (RCA120, PHA(E), DSA, BPL, PWM, Jacalin) were higher, and five lectins (NPA, GNA, HHL, TxLC-I, EEL) were lower. Finally, in the case of ED, seven lectins (AAL, PHA(E), DSA, LEL, Jacalin, WGA) interact higher, and other seven lectins (SNA, SSA, TJA-I, NPA, GNA, HHL, EEL) got lower.

Using those digitized lectin intensities, we performed clustering analysis of these six subjects by NIA Array Analysis (http://lgsun.grc.nia.nih.gov/ANOVA/). Fig. 4 shows the clustering results. It is easily appreciated that (1) two PBLs behave very similar manners, (2) C8166 and

ATL4 form the same cluster, (3) ED, non-Tax and dispersed, distinctive from other three cell lines, showed larger distance from others, and (4) ATL9, low-Tax and moderate cell aggregation, positioned between ED and C8166, ATL4.

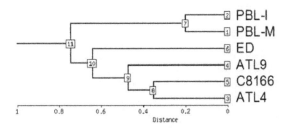

Figure 4. Hierarchical clustering of the six subject's glycan profiles

These results indicated that lectin microarray analysis detected the subtle differences of glycan profiles which synchronized with Tax-expression, NF-κB activation and cellular aggregation behaviors and this novel method would provide a diagnostic criteria for ATL's pathological development.

Acknowledgements

We thank Dr. M. Tomita for providing the opportunity of review article. Ms. E. Ikebe provided all the results presented in this article. E.I. is a research fellow of the Okinawa Science and Technology Promotion Center. This study is supported in part by grants from Japan Science and Technology Agency; Ministry of Education, Culture, Sports, Science, and Technology; Ministry of Economy, Trade and Industry; Okinawa Science and Technology Promotion Center; Miyazaki Prefectural Industrial Support Foundation; and the Research fund of Hita Tenryosui Co. Ltd.

Author details

Hidekatsu Iha[1*] and Masao Yamada[2]

*Address all correspondence to: hiha@oita-u.ac.jp

1 Department of Microbiology, Oita University Faculty of Medicine, Idaigaoka, Hasama, Yufu, Japan

2 GP Biosciences Ltd, -3-3, Azamino-minami, Aoba-ku, Yokohama, Japan

References

[1]   Amano, M, Setoyama, M, Grant, A, & Kerdel, F. A. Int J Dermatol. (2011). Human T-
      lymphotropic virus 1 (HTLV-1) infection-dermatological implications., 50(8), 915-920.

[2]   Andrisani, O, & Dixon, J. E. J Biol Chem. (1990). Identification and purification of a
      novel 120-kDa protein that recognizes the cAMP-responsive element., 265, 3212-3218.

[3]   Bazarbachi, A, & Plumelle, Y. Carlos Ramos J, Tortevoye P, Otrock Z, Taylor G, Ges-
      sain A, Harrington W, Panelatti G, Hermine O. J Clin Oncol. (2010). Meta-analysis on
      the use of zidovudine and interferon-alfa in adult T-cell leukemia/lymphoma show-
      ing improved survival in the leukemic subtypes., 28, 4177-4183.

[4]   Baum, P. R, & Gayle, R. B. rd, Ramsdell F, Srinivasan S, Sorensen RA, Watson ML,
      Seldin MF, Baker E, Sutherland GR, Clifford KN, et al. EMBO J. (1994). Molecular
      characterization of murine and human OX40/OX40 ligand systems: identification of a
      human OX40 ligand as the HTLV-1-regulated protein gp34., 13, 3992-4001.

[5]   Dnistrian, A. M, & Schwartz, M. K. Clin Chem. (1981). Plasma lipid-bound sialic acid
      and carcinoembryonic antigen in cancer patients., 27, 1737-1739.

[6]   Feizi, T. Nature. (1985). Demonstration by monoclonal antibodies that carbohydrate
      structures of glycoproteins and glycolipids are onco-developmental antigens., 314,
      53-57.

[7]   Fujii, M, Niki, T, Mori, T, Matsuda, T, Matsui, M, Nomura, N, & Seiki, M. Oncogene.
      (1991). HTLV-1 Tax induces expression of various immediate early serum responsive
      genes., 6, 1023-1029.

[8]   Fujisawa, J, Seiki, M, Kiyokawa, T, & Yoshida, M. Proc Natl Acad Sci U S A. (1985).
      Functional activation of the long terminal repeat of human T-cell leukemia virus type
      I by a trans-acting factor., 82, 2277-2281.

[9]   Fukuda, M. Cancer Res. (1996). Possible roles of tumor-associated carbohydrate anti-
      gens., 56, 2237-2244.

[10] Fuster, M. M, & Esko, J. D. Nat Rev Cancer. (2005). The sweet and sour of cancer: gly-
      cans as novel therapeutic targets., 5, 526-242.

[11] Gagneux, P, & Varki, A. Glycobiology. (1999). Evolutionary considerations in relat-
      ing oligosaccharide diversity to biological function., 9, 747-755.

[12] Gallo, R. C, Mann, D, Broder, S, Ruscetti, F. W, Maeda, M, Kalyanaraman, V. S, &
      Robert-guroff, M. Reitz MS Jr. Proc Natl Acad Sci U S A. (1982). Human T-cell leuke-
      mia-lymphoma virus (HTLV) is in T but not B lymphocytes from a patient with cuta-
      neous T-cell lymphoma., 79, 5680-5683.

[13] Gaudray, G, Gachon, F, Basbous, J, Biard-piechaczyk, M, Devaux, C, & Mesnard, J.
      M. J Virol. (2002). The complementary strand of the human T-cell leukemia virus

type 1 RNA genome encodes a bZIP transcription factor that down-regulates viral transcription., 76, 12813-12822.

[14] Gonçalves, D. U, Proietti, F. A, Ribas, J. G, Araújo, M. G, Pinheiro, S. R, Guedes, A. C, & Carneiro-proietti, A. B. Clin Microbiol Rev. (2010). Epidemiology, treatment, and prevention of human T-cell leukemia virus type 1-associated diseases., 23, 577-589.

[15] Hakomori, S, & Kannagi, R. J Natl Cancer Inst. (1983). Glycosphingolipids as tumor-associated and differentiation markers., 71, 231-251.

[16] Himes, S. R, Coles, L. S, Katsikeros, R, Lang, R. K, & Shannon, M. F. Oncogene. (1993). HTLV-1 tax activation of the GM-CSF and G-CSF promoters requires the interaction of NF-kB with other transcription factor families., 8, 3189-3197.

[17] Hinuma, Y, Nagata, K, Hanaoka, M, Nakai, M, Matsumoto, T, Kinoshita, K. I, Shirakawa, S, & Miyoshi, I. Proc Natl Acad Sci U S A. (1981). Adult T-cell leukemia: antigen in an ATL cell line and detection of antibodies to the antigen in human sera., 78, 6476-680.

[18] Hynes, R. O, & Naba, A. Cold Spring Harb Perspect Biol. (2012). 4:a004903. Overview of the matrisome--an inventory of extracellular matrix constituents and functions.

[19] Inose, M, Higuchi, I, Yoshimine, K, Suehara, M, Izumo, S, Arimura, K, & Osame, M. J Neurol Sci. (1992). Pathological changes in skeletal muscle in HTLV-I-associated myelopathy., 110, 73-78.

[20] Iwanaga, M, Watanabe, T, Utsunomiya, A, Okayama, A, Uchimaru, K, Koh, K. R, Ogata, M, Kikuchi, H, Sagara, Y, Uozumi, K, Mochizuki, M, Tsukasaki, K, Saburi, Y, Yamamura, M, Tanaka, J, Moriuchi, Y, Hino, S, & Kamihira, S. Yamaguchi K; Joint Study on Predisposing Factors of ATL Development investigators. Blood. (2010). Aug; Human T-cell leukemia virus type I (HTLV-1) proviral load and disease progression in asymptomatic HTLV-1 carriers: a nationwide prospective study in Japan., 116, 1211-1219.

[21] Kannagi, R, Izawa, M, Koike, T, Miyazaki, K, & Kimura, N. Cancer Sci. (2004). Carbohydrate-mediated cell adhesion in cancer metastasis and angiogenesis., 95, 377-384.

[22] Kawai, H, Kashiwagi, S, Sano, Y, Inui, T, & Saito, S. Rinsho Shinkeigaku. (1991). HTLV-I associated myelopathy with Hashimoto's thyroiditis--a report of two cases., 31, 648-652.

[23] Kimura, I, Tsubota, T, Ueda, N, Tada, S, Yoshimoto, S, Sogawa, J, Shiraishi, T, Tamaki, T, Ueno, K, Fujita, T, et al. Nihon Kyobu Shikkan Gakkai Zasshi. (1989). Six cases of HTLV-I associated bronchiolo-alveolar disorder (HABA)., 27, 1074-1081.

[24] Kuno, A, Uchiyama, N, Ebe, K-K. u. n. o S, Takashima, Y, Yamada, S, & Hirabayashi, M. J. Nature Methods, 2005; Evanescent-field fluorescence-assisted lectin microarray: a new strategy for glycan profiling. La Grenade L, Hanchard B, Fletcher V, Cranston

B, Blattner W. Lancet. (1990). Infective dermatitis of Jamaican children: a marker for HTLV-I infection., 2, 851-856.

[25] Manns, A, & Blattner, W. A. Transfusion. (1991). The epidemiology of the human T-cell lymphotrophic virus type I and type II: etiologic role in human disease., 31, 67-75.

[26] Mochizuki, M, Watanabe, T, Yamaguchi, K, Takatsuki, K, Yoshimura, K, Shirao, M, Nakashima, S, Mori, S, Araki, S, & Miyata, N. Jpn J Cancer Res. (1992). HTLV-I uveitis: a distinct clinical entity caused by HTLV-I., 83, 236-239.

[27] Nakano, K, & Watanabe, T. Nihon Rinsho. (2012). Apr; Current status and problems of anti-HTLV-1 drug development., 70(4), 671-5.

[28] Nasr, R, El Hajj, H, Kfoury, Y, De Thé, H, Hermine, O, & Bazarbachi, A. Viruses. (2011). Controversies in targeted therapy of adult T cell leukemia/lymphoma: ON target or OFF target effects?, 3, 750-769.

[29] Nishioka, K, Maruyama, I, Sato, K, Kitajima, I, Nakajima, Y, & Osame, M. Lancet. (1989). Feb 25;1(8635):441 Chronic inflammatory arthropathy associated with HTLV-I.

[30] Olière, S, Douville, R, Sze, A, Belgnaoui, S. M, & Hiscott, J. Cytokine Growth Factor Rev. (2011). Modulation of innate immune responses during human T-cell leukemia virus (HTLV-1) pathogenesis., 22, 197-210.

[31] Osame, M, Usuku, K, Izumo, S, Ijichi, N, Amitani, H, Igata, A, Matsumoto, M, & Tara, M. Lancet. (1986). HTLV-I associated myelopathy, a new clinical entity., 1(8488), 1031-1032.

[32] Proietti, F. A, Carneiro-proietti, A. B, Catalan-soares, B. C, & Murphy, E. L. Oncogene. (2005). Global epidemiology of HTLV-I infection and associated diseases., 24, 6058-6068.

[33] Rademacher, T. W, Parekh, R. B, & Dwek, R. A. Annu. Rev. Biochem. (1988). Glycobiology., 57, 785-838.

[34] Ruben, S, Poteat, H, Tan, T. H, Kawakami, K, Roeder, R, Haseltine, W, & Rosen, C. A. Science. (1988). Cellular transcription factors and regulation of IL-2 receptor gene expression by HTLV-I tax gene product., 241, 89-92.

[35] Sanada, I, Kawano, F, Tsukamoto, A, & Kiyokawa, T. Rinsho Ketsueki. (1999). Adult T-cell leukemia with elevated serum hyaluronic acid levels paralleling disease activity., 40, 51-54.

[36] Sasaki, H, Nishikata, I, Shiraga, T, Akamatsu, E, Fukami, T, Hidaka, T, Kubuki, Y, Okayama, A, Hamada, K, Okabe, H, Murakami, Y, Tsubouchi, H, & Morishita, K. Blood. (2005). Overexpression of a cell adhesion molecule, TSLC1, as a possible molecular marker for acute-type adult T-cell leukemia., 105, 1204-1213.

[37] Satou, Y, Yasunaga, J, Zhao, T, Yoshida, M, Miyazato, P, Takai, K, Shimizu, K, Ohshi-ma, K, Green, P. L, Ohkura, N, Yamaguchi, T, Ono, M, Sakaguchi, S, & Matsuoka, M. PLoS Pathog. (2011). e1001274 HTLV-1 bZIP factor induces T-cell lymphoma and systemic inflammation in vivo.

[38] Sharon, N, & Lis, H. Sci. Am. (1993). Carbohydrates in cell recognition., 268, 82-89.

[39] Shimoyama, M. Br J Haematol. (1991). Diagnostic criteria and classification of clinical subtypes of adult T-cell leukaemia-lymphoma. A report from the Lymphoma Study Group (1984-87)., 79, 428-437.

[40] Sonoda, S, Li, H. C, & Tajima, K. Cancer Sci. (2011). Ethnoepidemiology of HTLV-1 related diseases: ethnic determinants of HTLV-1 susceptibility and its worldwide dis-persal., 102, 295-301.

[41] Sowa, J. M. J Rheumatol. (1992). Human T lymphotropic virus I, myelopathy, poly-myositis and synovitis: an expanding rheumatic spectrum., 19, 316-318.

[42] Teshigawara, K, Maeda, M, Nishino, K, Nikaido, T, Uchiyama, T, Tsudo, M, Wano, Y, & Yodoi, J. J Mol Cell Immunol. (1985). Adult T leukemia cells produce a lympho-kine that augments interleukin 2 receptor expression., 2, 17-26.

[43] Theocharis, A. D, Skandalis, S. S, Tzanakakis, G. N, Karamanos, N. K, & Febs, J. (2010). Proteoglycans in health and disease: novel roles for proteoglycans in malig-nancy and their pharmacological targeting., 277, 3904-3923.

[44] Tsukasaki, K. Hematology. (2012). Suppl 1:S Adult T-cell leukemia-lymphoma., 32-35.

[45] Tsukasaki, K, Hermine, O, Bazarbachi, A, Ratner, L, & Ramos, J. C. Harrington W Jr, O'Mahony D, Janik JE, Bittencourt AL, Taylor GP, Yamaguchi K, Utsunomiya A, To-binai K, Watanabe T. J Clin Oncol. (2009). Definition, prognostic factors, treatment, and response criteria of adult T-cell leukemia-lymphoma: a proposal from an inter-national consensus meeting., 27, 453-459.

[46] Varki, A. Glycobiology. (1993). Biological roles of oligosaccharides: All of the theories are correct., 3, 97-130.

[47] Varki, A, & Faseb, J. (1997). Sialic acids as ligands in recognition phenomena., 11, 248-255.

[48] Van Beek, W. P, Smets, L. A, & Emmelot, P. Nature. (1975). Changed surface glyco-protein as a marker of malignancy in human leukaemic cells., 253(5491), 457-460.

[49] Xu, Y. L, Adya, N, Siores, E, Gao, Q. S, & Giam, C. Z. J Biol Chem. (1990). Cellular factors involved in transcription and Tax-mediated trans-activation directed by the TGACGT motifs in human T-cell leukemia virus type I promoter., 265, 20285-20292.

[50] Yamagishi, M, Nakano, K, Miyake, A, Yamochi, T, Kagami, Y, Tsutsumi, A, Matsuda, Y, Sato-otsubo, A, Muto, S, Utsunomiya, A, Yamaguchi, K, Uchimaru, K, Ogawa, S,

& Watanabe, T. Cancer Cell. (2012). Polycomb-mediated loss of miR-31 activates NIK-dependent NF-κB pathway in adult T cell leukemia and other cancers., 21, 121-135.

[51] Yamaoka, S, Courtois, G, Bessia, C, Whiteside, S. T, Weil, R, Agou, F, Kirk, H. E, Kay, R. J, & Israël, A. Cell. (1998). Complementation cloning of NEMO, a component of the IkappaB kinase complex essential for NF-kappaB activation., 93, 1231-1240.

[52] Yeung, M. L, Yasunaga, J, Bennasser, Y, Dusetti, N, Harris, D, Ahmad, N, Matsuoka, M, & Jeang, K. T. Cancer Res. (2008). Roles for microRNAs, miR-93 and miR-130b, and tumor protein 53-induced nuclear protein 1 tumor suppressor in cell growth dysregulation by human T-cell lymphotrophic virus 1. US Patent 6,787,364 (2004), 68, 8976-8985.

Monoclonal Antibody Therapy of T-Cell Leukemia and Lymphoma

Tahir Latif and John C. Morris

Additional information is available at the end of the chapter

1. Introduction

T-cell leukemias and lymphomas are a heterogeneous group of uncommon tumors that account for 7-15% of lymphomas. [1] They represent approximately 6,500 new cases annually in the United States. Typically patients with malignant T-cell disorders present with high-grade lesions, advanced stage disease and have systemic or "B" symptoms at diagnosis. Until relatively recently these diseases were treated with the same anthracycline-based chemotherapy regimens used to treat B-cell lymphomas. With few exceptions, the outcomes are poorer with lower response rates, shorter times to progression, and shorter median survivals compared to B-cell lymphomas. A number of new agents have recently entered the clinic for the treatment of T-cell lymphomas. [2] These include the histone deacetylase inhibitors voronistat (Zolinza®) and romidepsin (Istodax®) approved for treatment of previously treated cutaneous T-cell lymphoma (CTCL), the antifolate, pralatrexate (Fotolyn®) indicated for the treatment of relapsed or resistant peripheral T-cell lymphoma (PTCL), and the immunotoxin brentuximab vedotin (Adcetris®) for the treatment of relapsed anaplastic large cell lymphoma (ALCL). These newer agents join a handful of drugs approved for the treatment of T-cell lymphomas including beraxotene (Targretin®) and the interleukin-2-diphtheria toxin fusion protein, denileukin diftitox (Ontak®).

The introduction of the chimerized anti-CD20 monoclonal antibody, rituximab (Rituxan®), was a major advance in the treatment of B-cell lymphoma improving the survival of patients with B-cell lymphoma. Unlike B-cell lymphomas no monoclonal antibody has received a similar indication for treatment of T-cell neoplasms. Presently an expanding number of antibodies targeting T-cells are being studied for the treatment of T-cell leukemia and lymphoma. The current status of monoclonal antibody therapy of T-cell leukemia and lymphoma will be the focus of this chapter.

Target Antigen	Description	Monoclonal Antibody
CD2	LFA-3 (CD58)	Slipizumab (MEDI-507)
CD3 (CD3ζ)	TcR signaling chain	muromonab-CD3 (Orthoclone®, OKT3)
CD4	TcR co-receptor	Zanolimumab (HuMax-CD4®)
CD5	Scavenger receptor family member	Anti-Leu1
		T101
CD25	IL-2 receptor α-subunit	Daclizumab (Zenapax®)
CD30	TNF receptor family member	Brentuximab vedotin (Adcetris®)
CD52	GPI-anchored glycoprotein	Alemtuzumab (Campath®)
CD122	β-subunit of the IL-2 and IL-15 receptor	Mik-β1
CCR4	Chemokine receptor-4	KW-0761

Table 1. Monoclonal antibodies for the treatment of T-cell leukemia and lyumphoma.

2. Characteristics of the ideal target for antibody-directed therapy

Delivering maximum therapeutic benefits with minimal or no toxicity have been the main objective of any therapeutic strategy including antibody therapy. The choice of therapeutic target for antibody therapy is one of the most important variables in achieving this goal. The ideal target for antibody-directed therapy should have following characteristics: Including restriction of the target antigen expression to malignant T-cells. Toxicity and unintended effects of a ubiquitously present target is a significant hindrance in development of antibody therapy, an ideal target should have its expression restricted to malignant T-cell or if the target is expressed on other hematopoietic cells, the loss of these cells or their function should not result in serious complications such as life-threatening immunosuppression. If the target is broadly expressed on other T-cells or hematopoietic cells, treatment will not only eliminate the tumor cells, it will also cause depletion of functional T-cells allowing reactivation or susceptibility to a variety of serious infections. Alemtuzumab (Campath®), a monoclonal antibody directed against CD52 is an effective therapy against B-cell chronic lymphocytic leukemia (CLL); however, since CD52 is also expressed on T-cells, treatment results in the depletion of both CD4+ and CD8+ T-cell populations and an increased risk of opportunistic infections. [3]

The target antigen ideally should be expressed at high density on the malignant T-cells. Most antibodies deliver their therapeutic effect by binding to the target on the cell surface, activating complement, antibody dependent cellular cytotoxicity (ADCC) or inducing signals activating apoptosis. The target receptor must be present in significant numbers on the cell surface to provide an adequate number of binding sites for the antibody. Down modulation and mutations in surface receptors can reduce binding of monoclonal antibodies interfering with their therapeutic efficacy. Modulation of surface receptor expression is an important physio-logical characteristic used by normal and malignant cells to control responsiveness to cytokines and other receptor ligands. For unmodified monoclonal antibodies ideally the antibody target should be non-modulating so that adequate target antigen is always available for antibody to exert its therapeutic effect. Modulating receptors internalize antibody-receptor complex leaving limited numbers of surface receptors causing relative resistance. Modulation; however, can be used to an advantage with immunotoxins and ligand-toxin fusion proteins that need internalization to exert their action, but in general, modulation reduces the effectiveness of monoclonal antibodies.

Other characteristics of the ideal monoclonal antibody should include that the targeting of the antigen by the antibody should not lead to serious side effects. In addition to their immuno-genicity causing infusion reactions and serum sickness, some monoclonal antibodies can stimulate the systemic release of inflammatory cytokines with serious consequences. A phase 1 dose-escalation trial testing an anti-CD28 monoclonal antibody (TGN1412) with 'super-agonist' effects on T-lymphocytes caused near-lethal acute systemic inflammation requiring hospitalization in six volunteers treated in a phase I study. [4]

3. Qualities of the antibody

Ideally the targeting antibody itself should be non-immunogenic, should act through several mechanisms of antitumor activity and have patient friendly dosing schedules and pharmaco-kinetics. [5] Current technologies has made it possible to engineer majority of antibodies in clinical use so that most of the molecule except for the receptor-binding domains is identical to that of a human antibody to reduce immunogenicity and the risk of neutralizing responses against the antibody. [6, 7]

3.1. Mechanism of action

Mechanisms of actions of monoclonal antibody action include induction of antibody-depend-ent cellular cytotoxicity (ADCC). A monoclonal antibody binds to its antigen target and recruits other components of cellular immune system such as NK cells, neutrophils, and eosinophils. These stimulated cells then attack and destroy the tumor cell. Some antibodies will directly bind to Fc receptors on effector cells such as macrophages and cytolytic T-cells causing destruction of the target cell through ADCC. [8]

Complement-mediated cytotoxicity (CMC) is another Fc-mediated mechanism of monoclonal antibody action. [9] It has been shown to play a roll in the antitumor activity of a number of antibodies including alemtuzumab. [10] In addition to CMC, complement fixation is also involved in inflammation, chemotaxis and opsonization, all of which may aid in tumor cell killing.

Monoclonal antibodies can also engage tumor cell surface receptors resulting into release of an apoptotic signal inducing tumor cell killing. Many of the cell surface markers including those of the tumor necrosis factor receptor (TNFR) family, Fas, and the receptors for TNF-related apoptosis-inducing ligand (TRAIL) when engaged by their ligand deliver an apoptotic signal promoting apoptosis. Monoclonal antibodies can mimic the physiologic ligand of these receptors and can agonistically bind to receptor family members eliciting apoptotic responses on engagement. [11] A number of monoclonal antibodies are known to induce tumor cell apoptosis at least partially through direct engagement of their target receptor including SGN-30 a chimeric anti-CD30 antibody, and alemtuzumab (anti-CD52). [12, 13]

Monoclonal antibodies can also hinder cell growth and regulation through blocking critical ligand-receptor interactions necessary for tumor survival and inducing receptor and down-modulation reducing pro-growth signaling. Daclizumab, the anti-CD25 antibody, exert its main cytotoxic effect by blocking the binding of IL-2 to its receptors depriving T-cells of a necessary growth factor resulting in cell death. [14]

3.2. Immunogenicity of monoclonal antibodies

3.2.1. Non-human monoclonal antibodies

Scientists have attempted to produce single specificity monoclonal antibodies for therapy for more than a century now. Despite early optimism the development of monoclonal antibodies as therapeutic modality remained elusive due to the immunogenicity of monoclonal antibodies. It was only with the introduction of hybridoma technology in 1975 the promise of selectively targeting cancers using monoclonal antibodies became a reality. [15] Early therapeutic monoclonal antibodies were derived primarily from rodents. These antibodies can be produced in large amounts and have greater specificity to their single antigenic determinant compared to polyclonal antisera used for therapeutic purposes. Unfortunately early attempts to use these mouse or rodent antibodies for therapeutic purposes were unsuccessful in large part due to the dissimilarity between the rodent and human immune systems. Initially developed non-human antibodies, as foreign glycoproteins, had several issues hindering their effectiveness and development. These rodent hybridoma-derived antibodies exhibited short *in vivo* half-lives, were highly immunogenic in man often inducing neutralizing human anti-mouse antibodies (HAMA), and they could not engage Fc receptors expressed on human effector cells resulting in their inability at inducing ADCC making them relatively weak cytotoxic agents. Due to the foreign protein sequences serum sickness, infusion reactions and anaphylaxis were also common with these antibodies. In addition, many of these early non-human monoclonal antibodies were not directed against cell surface targets that were accessible to the antibody limiting their efficacy. First FDA approved monoclonal antibody in 1986 for treatment of allogeneic transplant rejection, Muromonab-CD3 (Orthoclone® OKT3), an anti-CD3 monoclonal antibody, is a non-human monoclonal antibody. [16]

3.2.2. Chimerized antibodies

Rapid neutralization of therapeutic antibodies due to formation of immune complexes between the non-human monoclonal antibody and induced host antibodies can severely limit tumor response and may alter antibody distribution and binding resulting in undesired side effects. Engineering of non-human monoclonal antibodies with human constant domains, so called chimerized or humanized monoclonal antibodies, or the generation of fully human monoclonal antibodies using transgenic or phage display technology has helped overcome many of these issues of immunogenicity. [17-19]

Chimeric monoclonal antibodies are generated by linking the rodent light and heavy chain variable domains to the human immunoglobulin constant domains using recombinant DNA technology. [20] This results in an antibody that contains approximately 65% human sequences that exhibits reduced immunogenicity and an increased serum half-life. Although the immunogenicity of chimeric monoclonal antibodies is significantly reduced, they are occasionally still capable of eliciting a human anti-chimera response (HACA) in some patients.

3.2.3. Chimerized monoclonal antibodies

Second generation monoclonal antibodies were further improved by incorporating the six complementarity-determining regions (CDR) of the rodent antibody-antigen binding site onto a human IgG antibody framework. Further improvements in maintaining the structure of the antigen-binding site and high affinity binding to the target were made by incorporating small number of amino acids in the murine antibody not directly involved in the CDR. [21] Alemtuzumab is one such example. Although the binding between humanized antibodies and the dissociation constants (K_d) of humanized and the parental monoclonal antibody target is weaker than the murine parent, the differences between these are usually small enough to not be significant. [22, 23] Polymorphisms located in the constant regions, or to anti-idiotypic recognition of the variable domain can rarely result in human anti-human (HAHA) antibody responses. [24, 25]

3.2.4. Fully human monoclonal antibodies

To further enhance efficacy, "fully human" monoclonal antibodies have been generated using transgenic mice expressing human immunoglobulin genes. Vaccination of these mice using the desired antigen induces B-cells producing a fully human antibody by the mouse. Panitumumab (Vectibix®) an anti-EGFR monoclonal antibody [26], and ofatumumab (Azerra®), an anti-CD20 monoclonal antibody, were generated using such an approach. Phage display technology has also made it possible to develop fully human monoclonal antibody with significant clinical activity. Phage display techniques have the added benefit of also allowing the enhanced selection of therapeutically relevant features of antibodies. [27]

3.3. Fully human monoclonal antibodies

Most antibodies in clinical use exert their antitumor effect through direct antibody-mediated killing. In an effort to increase cytotoxic effect of monoclonal antibodies other modifications were made to enhance their affinity or cell toxicity by combining the antibody with a toxin or radioisotope.

The antibody Fc region mediates effector function and may be altered to augment binding to FcRIII, a stimulatory receptor and reduce binding to FcRII, an inhibitory receptor, to enhance

ADCC. One strategy is to engineer Fc portions that exhibit reduced fucose glycosylation. [28] Alternatively, the Fc region may be engineered to reduce or enhance CMC by substituting antibody isotypes such as IgG4 that exhibit little complement activation or Fc receptor binding. An additional interaction of the Fc region is with the neonatal receptor FcRn that is involved with immunoglobulin turnover. This receptor interacts with IgG Fc in a saturable and pH dependent manner, this allows FcRn to bind IgG from acidic endosomes generated during pinocytosis, and recycle the IgG back to the cell surface where it is released in the slightly basic pH of the blood. This allows for an extended antibody half-life. This approach holds much promise for favorably altering the pharmacokinetics of monoclonal antibodies ultimately leading to the potential for less frequent administration of these expensive treatments.

3.4. Immunotoxins

Immunotoxins are conjugations of monoclonal antibodies with toxins that result in highly specific cytotoxicity. In this approach it is desirable for the target antigen to be internalized upon antibody binding delivering the toxin into the cell. These toxins, often derived from bacteria or plants sources, are extremely potent. Bacterial toxins such as diphtheria toxin (DT) and *Pseudomonas* exotoxin A inhibit cellular protein synthesis by the irreversible ADP ribosy-lation of elongation factor-2 (EF-2), while plant toxins such as ricin inactivate ribosomes. [29] Disadvantages of this approach include the increased immunogenicity of most of these toxins because of their microbial or plant origins. In addition, many immunotoxin conjugates are non-specifically taken up by pinocytocysis by endothelial cell resulting in a vascular leak syndrome with edema and weight gain. In 2011, Brentuximab vendotin (Adcetris®), an immunotoxin composed of an anti-CD30 monoclonal antibody (SGN-30) and the potent anti-microtubule agent monomethylauristatin (MMAE) was approved for previously treated anaplastic large cell lymphoma and Hodgkin's lymphoma. [30] Denileukin difitox (Ontak®) approved for the treatment cutaneous T-cell lymphoma is often categorized as an immunotoxin; however, this agent is not antibody-based, but rather represents a fusion protein between the receptor binding domain of interleukin-2 and diphtheria toxin linked by short peptide sequence. [31]

3.5. Radioimmunotherapy

Radioimmunotherapy combines the specificity of monoclonal antibodies with the tumor killing effects of radiation, in theory sparing non-target cells from exposure to high doses of radiation. The choice of an appropriate antigen target and hence the specific monoclonal antibody is critical, as off target killing needs to be avoided. One consequence of this is the "bystander" or "cross-fire" effect, as radiation can also kill adjacent tumor cells that may not express the target antigen. The greatest clinical experience with radioimmunotherapy is in CD20-expressing lymphomas using radionuclides such as yttrium-90 (^{90}Y) and iodine-131 (^{131}I) labeled anti-CD20 monoclonal antibodies.

4. Antibody therapy for T-cell leukemias and lymphomas

4.1. Anti-CD2 antibodies

CD2 is a surface glycoprotein that plays a key role in lymphocyte adhesion and signaling. [32] It is expressed on human T-lymphocytes, natural killer (NK) cells, and thymocytes, and its stimulation results in T-cell activation and antigen co-stimulation. It also potentiates the physical interaction between T-cells and antigen presenting cells, as well as between T-cells and NK-cells. In the cell membrane, CD2 associates with the T-cell receptor (TcR) and appears to enhance CD3 signaling during low affinity interactions with the major histocompatibility complex (MHC) molecules enhancing class I and class II-restricted antigen recognition. [33]

Siplizumab is humanized IgG1 monoclonal antibodies that binds to CD2 and inhibits T-cell responses and induced severe T-cell lymphopenia. It has primarily been studied as treatment for refractory psoriasis and treatment for graft-versus-host disease occurring during allogeneic bone marrow transplant. It has shown to increase disease-free survival of mice inoculated with human MET-1 adult T-cell leukemia cells. [34] In a phase I/II trial [35], 29 patients with various T-cell malignancies including HTLV-1-associated adult T-cell leukemia, peripheral T-cell lymphoma, cutaneous T-cells lymphoma, T-cell chronic lympho-cytic leukemia, and T-cell large granular lymphocyte leukemia were treated with siplizu-mab. Twenty-eight patients experienced a marked decline in circulating CD4+ and CD8+ T-cells, and NK-cells and there were two complete and nine partial responses. Unfortunately, four patients (13.7%) developed Epstein-Barr virus-related B-cell lymphoproliferative disease (EBV-LPD). [36] This complication has significantly hindered the development of siplizumab. A Phase I trial of siplizumab combined with rituximab and dose-adjusted etoposide, prednisone, vincristine, cyclophosphamide and doxorubicin (EPOCH) for T- and NK cell lymphoma is currently ongoing at the National Cancer Institute, where the rituximab is used to prophylaxis against the risk of EBV-LPD.

4.2. Anti-CD3 antibodies

CD3 represents a series of intermediate molecular weight polypeptide chains (CD3γ, CD3δ, CD3ϵ and CDζ) closely associated with α and β-subunits of the T-cell receptor (TcR) that recognizes antigen-peptide epitopes presented by MHC molecules in a class-restricted manner. [37] The intracellular regions of the CD3-subunits represent the signaling domains of the TcR complex that mediates T-cell activation. CD3 is expressed on most T-cells throughout development and thus represents a pan-T-cell antigen. The vast majority of T-cell neoplasms express CD3, although its expression may be reduced or lost in some lesions. [38]

Muromonab-CD3 (Orthoclone®, OKT3; Janssen Pharmaceutica, Ltd.), a murine IgG$_{2a}$ monoclonal antibody directed against the 20 kDa CD3ζ-subunit is approved for the reversal of acute allograft rejection in patients undergoing cardiac, hepatic and renal transplants. [39] It has also been used for the depletion of T-cells from stem cell and bone marrow allog-rafts to treat or reduce the risk of serious GvHD. [40] Administration of muromonab-CD3 results in the rapid disappearance of CD3+ T-cells from the peripheral circulation and lymphoid tissue through complement-mediated lysis, ADCC, apoptosis and the re-direction of T-lymphocytes to other compartments. [41] Binding of muromonab-CD3 to its target receptor also stimulates TcR signaling, activation and proliferation of T-cells with increased expression of HLA-DR and CD25.

In one report, a patient with refractory T-cell acute lymphoblastic leukemia that received muromonab-CD3 experienced a dramatic, albeit transient decline in circulating lymphoblasts and a reduction in splenomegaly. [42] Muromonmab-CD3 therapy is made difficult because engagement of the antibody with CD3ζ increases TcR signaling and can result in the release of inflammatory cytokines that can cause life-threatening cytokine release syndrome. In addition, muromonab-CD3 is also mitogenic for T-cells and its use may risk increasing the proliferation of malignant T-cells. Muromonmab-CD3 therapy is also associated with profound suppression of cell-mediated immunity and increased risk of opportunistic infections and secondary malignancies including EBV-LPD, lymphoma, skin cancer and Kaposi's sarcoma.

4.3. Anti-CD4 antibodies

CD4 is a 55 kDa membrane glycoprotein with four immunoglobulin-like domains, a hydrophobic transmembrane domain and a long cytoplasmic tail. [43] CD4 acts as a co-receptor for the TcR complex. It is expressed on helper and regulatory T-cells, and it recognizes antigens presented by MHC class II molecules in association with the TCR. CD4 represents an attractive target since the majority of the post-thymic T-cell malignancies manifest a CD4+ phenotype.

In phase I study, seven CTCL patients were treated with a chimeric antibody composed of the IgG₁κ human constant regions and the mouse variable regions directed against CD4 (anti-Leu3a). [44] Patients were dosed in cohorts of 10, 20, 40 or 80 mg intravenously twice a week for three weeks. At the 80 mg dose, the antibody was detected in skin lesions and also coating circulating CD4+ T-cells in the peripheral blood; however, with no significant depletion of CD4+ cells was observed. In a second study, this group administered a single intravenous dose of another chimeric murine anti-CD4 monoclonal antibody, cM-T412 (Centocor, Inc.), to eight previously treated CTCL patients. [45] Following the antibody infusion there was a significant suppression of peripheral blood CD4+ cells in seven of eight patients. Seven patients responded and the median duration of response was 25 weeks. One patient developed a neutralizing anti-chimeric antibody response. Toxicity was grade 2 or less and usually manifested as infusion reactions, mayalgias, and rashes.

More recently, zanolimumab (HuMax-CD4®; Genmab, Inc.), a fully human IgG₁κ anti-CD4 monoclonal antibody was shown to deplete CD4+ T-cells from the skin, reduce dermal inflammatory infiltrates and induce remissions in psoriasis patients. [46] Zanolimumab was evaluated in two separate phase II trials in a total of 47 CTCL/Sezary syndrome patients. [47] Patients received between 280 and 980 mg weekly for up to 17 weeks. Zanolimumab resulted in a dose-dependent and profound CD4+ lymphocytopenia; however, the recovery of CD4+ cells. Overall 13 of 38 (34.2%) CTCL patients and 2 of 9 (22.2%) patients with Sezary cell leukemia responded to the antibody. Adverse events included nine infections attributed to therapy. In a second phase II study, 21 adult patients with relapsed or refractory CD4+ PTCL of non-cutaneous type were treated in a single-arm multicenter study, with weekly intravenous infusions of zanolimumab 980 mg for 12 weeks. [48]. Objective tumor responses were observed in 24% of the patients with two complete responses and three partial responses. In general, the drug was well tolerated with no major toxicity. Zanolimumab at a dose of 980 mg weekly demonstrated clinical activity and an acceptable safety profile in this poor-prognosis patient population, suggesting that the potential benefit combining zanolimumab with standard chemotherapy in the treatment of PTCL should be investigated.

4.4. Anti-CD5 antibodies

CD5 (Leu-1) is a 67 kDa cysteine-rich scavenger receptor family glycoprotein expressed on T-cells and the B1a subset of B-cells. [49, 50] CD5 acts as a co-receptor and appears to regulate the signaling strength of the TcR signaling response. It may also play a similar role in modulating B-cell receptor signaling. [51] Current evidence indicates that CD5 is a key regulator of immune tolerance. Two small clinical trials have examined the use of anti-CD5 antibodies in patients with T-cell lymphoma. In one trial, 7 patients with refractory Leu-1+ (CD5+) T-cell lymphoma, six with CTCL and one with PTCL, were treated with murine anti-Leu-1 monoclonal antibody at doses of 0.25 to 100 mg administered 2-3 times per week. [52] A decrease in circulating T-cells was observed. The decline in T-cells was short-lived with a return to baseline occurring within 24-48 hours. The target antigen demonstrated down-modulation suggesting that CD5 might be a less suitable target for an unmodified antibody strategy. Five short-lived responses were reported and not surprisingly the majority of patients treated developed neutralizing antibodies. In another trial, T101, a murine IgG2a anti-CD5 monoclonal antibody was administered to eight patients with CD5+ T-cell malignancies, four of which had CTCL. [53] Short-lived clinical improvements were noted in two CTCL patients. Again, the induction of neutralizing antibodies was limiting. More recent trials of CD5-targeted therapy have focused on treatment of B-cell-induced autoimmune diseases and purging of T-cells from bone marrow to prevent GvHD and have used immunotoxin conjugates of anti-CD5. [54-56]

4.5. Anti-CD25

CD25 (IL-2Rα) is the 55 kDa subunit of the interleukin-2 (IL-2) receptor, and plays a critical role mediating immune-modulatory function of IL-2 in the activation of T- and B-lymphocytes, NK-cells and macrophages. [57, 58]. Less than 5% of un-stimulated peripheral blood T-cells expresses the IL-2Rα; however, it is highly expressed on activated T-cells and on many B- and T-cell neoplasms such as ATL, ALCL, CTCL, hairy cell leukemia, and on the Reed-Sternberg cells of Hodgkin's lymphoma. [59]

In 1981, Uchiyama and coworkers generated murine anti-Tac that defined the human IL-2Rα (CD25). [60] Daclizumab (Zenapax®; Hoffmann-La Roche, Inc.) is a recombinant monoclonal antibody where murine antigen-binding regions of the anti-Tac molecule were joined to a human immunoglobulin framework, approximately 90% of the murine IgG$_{2a}$ has been replaced with a human IgG$_{1\kappa}$ sequence. [61] Daclizumab has the advantages of a low frequency neutralizing antibodies, a significantly prolonged serum half-life compared to murine anti-

Tac, and the ability to mediate ADCC through its humanized Fc-domain. [62] It inhibits IL-2-induced activation of T-cells and it is approved for the prophylaxis of renal allograft rejection in combination with other immunosuppressive drugs.

Daclizumab up to 8 mg/kg was administered to ATL patients in one phase I/II trial. [63] Cohorts of patients were treated with daclizumab 2 mg/kg on days 1 and 2, or 4, 6, or 8 mg/kg as a single intravenous dose every 2 or 3 weeks to complete six doses. Although Daclizumab showed modest clinical activity (2 partial response and 3 patients with improvement of their skin disease), flow cytometry analysis of the peripheral blood 72 hours after the first dose and at weeks 2, 5 and 14 showed that ≥95% saturation of IL-2Rα on circulating ATL cells could be achieved and maintained. In six patients that underwent lymph node fine needle aspiration, receptor saturation was documented in only half and it was not maintained suggesting that the impeded access of large antibody molecules into tumor is a potential blockade to receptor-directed therapy.

4.6. Anti-CD30 antibodies

CD30 is a cellular membrane protein member of the tumor necrosis factor receptor (TNFR) family expressed on activated T- and B-cells. It is highly expressed on HL Reed–Sternberg (RS) cells, in anaplastic large cell lymphoma (ALCL), embryonal carcinomas, and select subtypes of B-cell derived, non-Hodgkin's lymphomas and mature T-cell lymphomas. The immuno-toxin brentuximab vedotin (Adcetris®, SGN-35) was approved by the FDA in 2011 and became the first new treatment for HL in 30 years. Brentuximab vedotin is an antibody-drug conjugate between the antitubulin agent monomethylauristatin E (MMAE) and the anti-CD30 monoclonal antibody cAC10. Clinical studies with unconjugated anti-CD30 antibodies have shown disappointing clinical activity. [64] Objective responses were observed in 6% of patients with HL who were treated with MDX-060 and in none of those treated with cAC10 (SGN-30). However, the results of a pivotal phase II study of brentuximab vedotin in relapsed or refractory HL were impressive [65]. In this study, 102 patients with refractory or relapsed classical HL received brentuximab vedotin every 3 weeks for a median of 27 weeks. Almost all patients exhibited a reduction in tumor volume with 34% complete response and 40% partial response. A phase II multicenter trial evaluated the efficacy and safety of brentuximab vedotin in relapsed or refractory systemic anaplastic large-cell lymphoma (ALCL) patients as CD30 is uniformly expressed in ALCL. [66] Fifty-eight patients received brentuximab vedotin 1.8 mg/kg intravenously every 3 weeks and 50 patients (86%) achieved an objective response, 33 patients (57%) achieved a complete remission (median duration 13.2 months) and 17 patients (29%) achieved a partial remission. Grade 3 or 4 adverse events observed in ≥10% of patients were neutropenia (21%), thrombocytopenia (14%), and peripheral neuropathy (12%). Based on these studies, brentuximab vedotin received accelerated approval for the treatment of Hodgkin lymphoma that has relapsed after autologous stem cell transplant and for the management of relapsed ALCL. Currently multiple studies are evaluating combination of brentuximab vedotin combined with standard chemotherapy options in management of both newly diagnosed and relapsed refractory ALCL patients.

4.7. Alemtuzumab (anti-CD52)

CD52 is a glycosylphosphatidylinositol (GPI)-anchored antigen expressed at high density on normal and malignant T- and B-cells, NK cells, monocytes, macrophages, eosinophils and epithelial cells of the male genital tract. It is not expressed on hematopoietic stem cells, granulocytes, erythrocytes, platelets, or plasma cells. Alemtuzumab (Campath®) a humanized rat monoclonal antibody targeting CD52 was approved by FDA for the treatment of relapsed/ refractory B-cell chronic lymphocytic leukemia (CLL). [67] Due to the presence of CD52 on T-cells and the antibody's ability to activate several mechanisms of cell death including ADCC, CMC and apoptosis it is an attractive agent to study in T-cell malignancies.

T-cell prolymphocytic leukemia (T-PLL) carries a worse prognosis than CLL and has no established standard therapy and thus constituted a fitting model to study alemtuzumab. An initial trial in 39 T-PLL patients showed an overall response rate of 76%, including 60% complete responses to alemtuzumab. [68] A subsequent study reported the experience with alemtuzumab in 76 T-PLL patients. [69] The objective response rate was 51% with almost 40% patients achieving complete response with median response duration of 8.7 months. The most common treatment-related adverse events were acute infusion reactions. There were 2 treatment-related deaths, 15 infectious episodes in 10 patients during active treatment, and 8 patients experienced late-onset infections due to the long lasting lymphopenia associated with alemtuzumab treatment.

These promising results in T-PLL lead to additional trials of alemtuzumab in both cutaneous T-cell lymphoma and other systemic T-cell malignancies either as a single agent or combined with chemotherapy. Single agent alemtuzumab is active in a variety of T-cell malignancies; however, responses are not durable and the risks of immunosuppression and development of opportunistic infections in patients poses a significant problem. In a phase II trial, alemtuzumab was administered to 22 patients with advanced mycosis fungoides/Sézary syndrome (MF/ SS). The overall response rate was 55%, with 32% of patients achieving a complete remission. [70] Remarkably after treatment, Sézary cells were undetectable in blood in 6 of 7 (86%) SS patients and pruritis significantly improved in responding patients. Patients with erythroderma responded better than patients with thick plaque disease or skin tumors.

In a pilot study, 14 patients with heavily pretreated peripheral T-cell lymphoma (PTCL) that received alemtuzumab for a maximum of 12 weeks showed a response rate of 36%. [71] Toxicity included cytomegalovirus (CMV) reactivation in 6 patients, pulmonary aspergillosis in 2 patients, and pancytopenia in 4 patients. Another trial reported on the efficacy of the combination of alemtuzumab combined with cyclophosphamide, doxorubicin, vincristine and prednisone (CHOP) as initial therapy for 24 PTCL patients. [72] The overall complete response rate was 71% (17 patients) and 1 patient a had partial remission. Grade 4 neutropenia and CMV reactivation was frequent. JC virus reactivation, invasive pulmonary aspergillosis, staphylococcal sepsis and pneumonia were also seen. In a recently reported phase II trial by the Dutch-Belgian HOVON group, 20 T-cell lymphoma patients were treated with 30 mg of alemtuzumab three times per week with every two week CHOP for eight courses. [73] The overall response was 90% and the median overall survival and event-free survival were 27 and 10 months, respectively. Although alemtuzumab-intensified CHOP achieved a high number of responses, many patients ultimately still relapsed, and this treatment was associated with frequent serious infection-related adverse events.

The combination of intravenous alemtuzumab 30 mg three times weekly and weekly pentostatin 4 mg/m^2 was studied in 24 patients with a variety of T-cell leukemias and lymphomas. [74] This trial showed an overall response rate of 54% with 11 complete responses and median response duration was 19.5 months. As with other trials opportunistic infections due to severe T-cell dysfunction were common in spite of antimicrobial prophylaxis.

4.8. Anti-CD122 (Mik-β1) antibodies

CD122 (IL-2R/IL-15Rβ) is a 75 kDa glycoprotein that constitutes the β-subunit shared by the IL-2 and IL-15 receptors. During signal transduction, CD 122 and CD132, the common γ-chain of type I cytokine receptors, recruit janus kinase (JAK), that in turn activates the signal transducer and activator of transcription (STAT). Activated STAT transcription factors enhances specific gene expression after translocation to nucleus. T-cell large granular lymphocyte (T-LGL) leukemia commonly presents with anemia, neutropenia and less frequently thrombocytopenia. IL-2 and IL-15 can stimulate T-LGL and NK cells and it is thought that the clinical cytopenias seen in T-LGL leukemia are a result of the enhanced NK activity of the leukemic cells. The Mik-β1 antibody (anti-CD122), directed against the IL-2R/IL-15Rβ, can inhibit IL-15-mediated effects *in vitro*. [75]

In a phase I trial, 12 patients with T-LGL leukemia received the murine Mik-β1 antibody and showed no responses in terms of decreases in T-LGL cell counts or improvement in their cytopenias. [76] Greater than 95% saturation of CD122 on circulating T-LGLs was achieved in all patients and down-modulation of CD122 was observed in seven patients. The lack of response may be the result of the short half-life of the murine antibody. In addition, down-modulation of CD122 after binding of the antibody reduced the amount of the receptor on the surface of the LGL cells and might have impacted the efficacy of the Mik-β1 antibody. A phase I safety and pharmacokinetic study of the humanized form of the antibody, HuMik-β1, in T-LGL leukemia patients was recently completed, but the results are not available.

4.9. KW-0761 (anti-CCR4)

Chemokine receptor-4 (CCR4) is over expressed on several T-cell neoplasms in addition to its normal expression on T-helper type 2 and regulatory T-cells. [77]. KW-0761 is a humanized IgG1 monoclonal antibody with a defucosylated Fc region that markedly enhances ADCC due to its increased binding affinity to the Fcγ receptor on effector cells. [78]. In a Phase I trial in 16 patients with relapsed CCR4-positive adult T-cell leukemia/lymphoma (ATL) or PTCL received KW-0761 once a week for 4 weeks by intravenous infusion. Toxicities included infusion reactions and skin rashes. The objective response rate was 31% with two complete and three partial responses. [79] Recently a multicenter phase II study conducted on 28 patients with relapsed ATL showed overall objective response rate of 50%, including eight complete responses, with a median progression-free and overall survival of 5.2 and 13.7 months, respectively. [80] The most common adverse events were infusion reactions (89%) and skin rashes (63%), which were manageable and reversible in all cases. Based on these results, a multicenter randomized phase II trial is ongoing comparing KW-0761 with standard second-line therapy according to investigator's choice of pralatrexate, gemcitabine and oxaliplatin, or dexamethasone, cisplatin and cytarabine in previously treated relapsed ATL.

5. Conclusions

T-cell leukemias and lymphomas represent a heterogeneous group of uncommon diseases that often present with advanced stage disease and systemic symptoms. Historically they have been treated with combination chemotherapy similar to high-grade B-cell lymphomas; however, outcomes have been poorer. One of the reasons for this may be the lack of effective monoclonal antibody therapy for these diseases comparable to that of rituximab for the B-cell disorders. A number of antibodies targeting surface receptors on T-cells are being clinically studied. Alemtuzumab, a CD52-directed monoclonal antibody has demonstrated antitumor activity as a single agent and in combination with chemotherapy, but with increased risk of serious opportunistic infections. Zanolimumab and KW-0761 directed against CD4 and CCR4 expressed on T-cells, have also show an activity against CTCL and ATL, respectively and are being studied in ongoing clinical trials and offer hope for the future for patients with T-cell malignancies.

Author details

Tahir Latif and John C. Morris*

*Address all correspondence to: morri2j7@ucmail.uc.edu

Division of Hematology-Oncology, Department of Medicine, University of Cincinnati, Cincinnati, OH, USA

References

[1] Savage, KJ. Update: peripheral T-cell lymphomasCurr Hematol Malig Rep. (2011). , 6, 222-30.

[2] Savage, KJ. Therapies for peripheral T-cell lymphomas. Hematology Am Soc Hematol Educ Program. (2011). , 2011, 515-24.

[3] Nosari, A, Montillo, M, & Morra, E. Infectious toxicity using alemtuzumab. Haematologica. (2004). , 89, 1414-9.

[4] Suntharalingam, G, Perry, MR, Ward, S, Brett, SJ, Castello-cortes, A, Brunner, MD, & Panoskaltsis, N. Cytokine storm in a phase I trial of the anti-CD28 monoclonal antibody TGN1412. N. Engl. J. Med. (2006). , 355, 1018-28.

[5] Golay, J, & Introna, M. Mechanism of action of therapeutic monoclonal antibodies: Promises and pitfalls of in vitro and in vivo assays. Arch Biochem Biophys. (2012). , 256, 146-53.

[6] Mascelli, MA, Zhou, H, Sweet, R, Getsy, J, Davis, HM, Graham, M, & Abernethy, D. Molecular, biologic, and pharmacokinetic properties of monoclonal antibodies: impact of these parameters on early clinical development. J Clin Pharmacol. (2007). , 47, 553-65.

[7] Lonberg, N. Human antibodies from transgenic animals. Nat Biotechnol. (2005). , 23, 1117-25.

[8] Zhang, M, Zhang, Z, Garmestani, K, Goldman, CK, Ravetch, JV, Brechbiel, MW, Carrasquillo, JA, & Waldmann, TA. Activating Fc receptors are required for antitumor efficacy of the antibodies directed toward CD25 in a murine model of adult T-cell leukemia. Cancer Res. (2004). , 64, 5825-9.

[9] Di Gaetano, N, Cittera, E, Nota, R, Vecchi, A, Grieco, V, Scanziani, E, Botto, M, Introna, M, & Golay, J. Complement activation determines the therapeutic activity of rituximab in vivo. J Immunol 2003

[10] Hale, G, Bright, S, Chumbley, G, Hoang, T, Metcalf, D, Munro, AJ, & Waldmann, H. Removal of T cells from bone marrow for transplantation: a monoclonal antilymphocyte antibody that fixes human complement. Blood. (1983). , 62, 873-82.

[11] Takeda, K, Stagg, J, Yagita, H, Okumura, K, & Smyth, MJ. Targeting death-inducing receptors in cancer therapy. Oncogene (2007). , 26, 3745-57.

[12] Lowenstein, H, Shah, A, Chant, A, & Khan, A. Different mechanisms of Campath-1H-mediated depletion for CD4 and CD8 T cells in peripheral blood.Transpl Int. (2006). , 19, 927-36.

[13] Rowan, W, Tite, J, Topley, P, & Brett, SJ. Cross-linking of the CAMPATH-1 antigen (CD52) mediates growth inhibition in human B- and T-lymphoma cell lines, and subsequent emergence of CD52-deficient cells. Immunology (1998). , 95, 427-36.

[14] Tkaczuk, J, Yu, CL, Baksh, S, Milford, EL, Carpenter, CB, Burakoff, SJ, & Mckay, DB. Effect of anti-IL-2Ralpha antibody on IL-2-induced Jak/STAT signaling. Am J Transplant. (2002). , 2, 31-40.

[15] Kohler, G, & Milstein, C. Continuous cultures of fused cells secreting antibody of predefined specificity. Nature. (1975). , 256, 495-7.

[16] Goldstein, G, Norman, DJ, Shield, CF, Kreis, H, Burdick, J, Flye, MW, Rivolta, E, Starzl, T, & Monaco, A. OKT3 monoclonal antibody reversal of acute renal allograft

rejection unresponsive to conventional immunosuppressive treatments. Prog Clin Biol Res. (1986). , 224, 239-49.

[17] Hudson, PJ, & Souriau, C. Engineered antibodies. Nat Med. (2003).

[18] Riechmann, L, Clark, M, Waldmann, H, & Winter, G. Reshaping human antibodies for therapy. Nature. (1988). , 332, 323-27.

[19] Winter, G, & Milstein, C. Man-made antibodies. Nature. (1991).

[20] Morrison, SL, Johnson, MJ, Herzenberg, LA, & Oi VT. Chimeric human antibody molecules: mouse antigen-binding domains with human constant region domains. Proc Natl Acad Sci USA. (1984). , 81, 6851-5.

[21] Queen, C, Schneider, WP, Selick, HE, Payne, PW, Landolfi, NF, Duncan, JF, Avdalovic, NM, Levitt, M, Junghans, RP, & Waldmann, TA. A humanized antibody that binds to the interleukin 2 receptor. Proc Natl Acad Sci USA. (1989). , 86, 10029-33.

[22] Presta, LG, Lahr, SJ, Shields, RL, Porter, JP, Gorman, CM, Fendly, BM, & Jardieu, PM. Humanization of an antibody directed against IgE. J Immunol. (1993). , 151, 2623-32.

[23] Carter, P, Presta, L, Gorman, CM, Ridgway, JB, Henner, D, Wong, WL, Rowland, AM, Kotts, C, Carver, ME, & Shepard, HM. Humanization of an anti-antibody for human cancer therapy. Proc Natl Acad Sci USA. (1992). , 185HER2.

[24] Aarden, L, Ruuls, SR, & Wolbink, G. Immunogenicity of anti-tumor necrosis factor antibodies-toward improved methods of anti-antibody measurement. Curr Opin Immunol. (2008). , 20, 431-5.

[25] Ritter, G, Cohen, LS, Williams, C, Jr., Richards, EC, Old, LJ, & Welt, S. Serological analysis of human anti-human antibody responses in colon cancer patients treated with repeated doses of humanized monoclonal antibody A33. Cancer Res. (2001). , 61, 6851-9.

[26] Jakobovits, A, Amado, RG, Yang, X, Roskos, L, & Schwab, G. From XenoMouse technology to panitumumab, the first fully human antibody product from transgenic mice. Nat Biotechnol. (2007). , 25, 1134-43.

[27] Hoogenboom, HR. Selecting and screening recombinant antibody libraries. Nat Biotechnol. (2005). , 23, 1105-16.

[28] Shinkawa, T, Nakamura, K, Yamane, N, Shoji-Hosaka, E, Kanda, Y, Sakurada, M, Uchida, K, Anazawa, H, Satoh, M, Yamasaki, M, Hanai, N, & Shitara, K. The absence of fucose but not the presence of galactose or bisecting N-acetylglucosamine of human IgG1 complex-type oligosaccharides shows the critical role of enhancing antibody-dependent cellular cytotoxicity. J Biol Chem. (2003). , 278, 3466-73.

[29] Kreitman. RJ. Recombinant toxins for the treatment of cancerCurr Opin Mol Ther (2003).

[30] Wahl, AF, Klussman, K, Thompson, JD, Chen, JH, Francisco, LV, Risdon, G, Chace, DF, Siegall, CB, & Francisco, JA. The anti-CD30 monoclonal antibody SGN-30 promotes growth arrest and DNA fragmentation in vitro and affects antitumor activity in models of Hodgkin's disease. Cancer Res. (2002). , 62, 3736-42.

[31] Olsen, E, Duvic, M, Frankel, A, Kim, Y, Martin, A, Vonderheid, E, Jegasothy, B, Wood, G, Gordon, M, Heald, P, Oseroff, A, Pinter-Brown, L, Bowen, G, Kuzel, T, Fivenson, D, Foss, F, Glode, M, Molina, A, Knobler, E, Stewart, S, Cooper, K, Stevens, S, Craig, F, Reuben, J, Bacha, P, & Nichols, J. Pivotal phase III trial of two dose levels of denileukin diftitox for the treatment of cutaneous T-cell lymphoma. J Clin Oncol. (2001). , 19, 376-88.

[32] Selvaraj, P, Plunkett, ML, Dustin, M, Sanders, ME, Shaw, S, & Springer, TA. The T lymphocyte glycoprotein CD2 binds the cell surface ligand LFA-3. Nature. (1987). , 326, 400-3.

[33] Moingeon, PE, Lucich, JL, Stebbins, CC, Recny, MA, Wallner, BP, Koyasu, S, & Reinherz, EL. Complementary roles for CD2 and LFA-1 adhesion pathways during T cell activation. Eur J Immunol. (1991). , 21, 605-10.

[34] Zhang, Z, Zhang, M, Ravetch, JV, Goldman, C, & Waldmann, TA. Effective therapy for a murine model of adult T-cell leukemia with the humanized anti-CD2 monoclonal antibody, MEDI-507. Blood. (2003). , 102, 284-8.

[35] Janik, JE, Morris, JC, Stetler-Stevenson, M, Gao, WW, O'Hagan, D, Moses, LS, Taylor, M. McEwen, C, Hammershaimb, LD, & Waldmann, TA. Phase I trial of siplizumab in CD2-positive lymphoproliferative disease. J Clin Oncol, ASCO Annual Proc. 23, 2005, 2533.

[36] O'Mahony, D, Morris, JC, Stetler-Stevenson, M, Matthews, H, Brown, MR, Fleisher, T, Pittaluga, S, Raffeld, M, Albert, PS, Reitsma, D, Kaucic, K, Hammershaimb, LD, Waldmann, TA, & Janik, JE. EBV-related lymphoproliferative disease complicating therapy with the anti-CD2 monoclonal antibody, siplizumab, in patients with T-cell malignancies. Clin Cancer Res. (2009)., 15, 2514-22.

[37] Garcia, KC, & Adams, EJ. How the T cell receptor sees antigen--a structural view. Cell. (2005). , 122, 333-6.

[38] Ohno, T, Yamaguchi, M, Oka, K, Miwa, H, Kita, K, & Shirakawa, S. Frequent expression of CD3 epsilon in CD3 (Leu 4)-negative nasal T-cell lymphomas. Leukemia. (1995). , 9, 44-52.

[39] Kirk, AD. Induction immunosuppression. Transplantation. (2006). , 82, 593-602.

[40] Knop, S, Hebart, H, Gratwohl, A, Kliem, C, Faul, C, Holler, E, Apperley, J, Kolb, HJ, Schaefer, A, Niederwieser, D, & Einsele, H. Treatment of steroid-resistant acute GVHD with OKT3 and high-dose steroids results in better disease control and lower incidence of infectious complications when compared to high-dose steroids alone: a

randomized multicenter trial by the EBMT Chronic Leukemia Working Party. Leukemia. (2007). , 21, 1830-3.

[41] Chatenoud, L. CD3-specific antibody-induced active tolerance: from bench to bedside. Nat Rev Immunol. (2003)., 3,123-32.

[42] Gramatzki, M, Burger, R, Strobel, G, Trautmann, U, Bartram, CR, Helm, G, Horneff, G, Alsalameh, S, Jonker, M, Gebhart, E, et al. Therapy with OKT3 monoclonal antibody in refractory T cell acute lymphoblastic leukemia induces interleukin-2 responsiveness. Leukemia. (1995). , 9, 382-90.

[43] Leahy, DJ. A structural view of CD4 and CD8. FASEB J. (1995)., 9, 17-25.

[44] Knox, S, Hoppe, RT, Maloney, D, Gibbs, I, Fowler, S, Marquez, C, Cornbleet, PJ, & Levy, R. Treatment of cutaneous T-cell lymphoma with chimeric anti-CD4 monoclonal antibody. Blood. (1996). , 87, 893-9.

[45] Knox, SJ, Levy, R, Hodgkinson, S, Bell, R, Brown, S, Wood, GS, Hoppe, R, Abel, EA, Steinman, L, Berger, RG, Gaiser, C, Young, G, Bindl, J, Hanham, A, & Reichert, T. Observations on the effect of chimeric anti-CD4 monoclonal antibody in patients with mycosis fungoides. Blood. (1991). , 77, 20-30.

[46] Skov, L, Kragballe, K, Zachariae, C, Obitz, ER, Holm, EA, Jemec, GB, Sølvsten, H, Ibsen, HH, Knudsen, L, Jensen, P, Petersen, JH, Menné, T, & Baadsgaard, O. HuMax-CD4: a fully human monoclonal anti-CD4 antibody for the treatment of psoriasis vulgaris. Arch Dermatol. (2003). , 139, 1433-9.

[47] Kim, YH, Duvic, M, Obitz, E, Gniadecki, R, Iversen, L, Osterborg, A, Whittaker, S, Illidge, TM, Schwarz, T, Kaufmann, R, Cooper, K, Knudsen, KM, Lisby, S, Baadsgaard, O, & Knox, SJ. Clinical efficacy of zanolimumab (HuMax-CD4): two phase 2 studies in refractory cutaneous T-cell lymphoma. Blood. (2007). , 109, 4655-62.

[48] d'Amore, F, Radford, J, Relander, T, Jerkeman, M, Tilly, H, Osterborg, A, Morschhauser, F, Gramatzki, M, Dreyling, M, Bang, B, & Hagberg, H. II trial of zanolimumab (HuMax-CD4) in relapsed or refractory non-cutaneous peripheral T cell lymphoma. Br J Haematol. (2010). , 150, 565-73.

[49] Ledbetter, JA, Rouse, RV, Micklem, HS, & Herzenberg, LA. T cell subsets defined by expression of Lyt-1,2,3 and Thy-1 antigens. Two-parameter immunofluorescence and cytotoxicity analysis with monoclonal antibodies modifies current views. J Exp Med. (1980). , 152, 280-95.

[50] Lozano, F, Simarro, M, Calvo, J, Vilà, JM, Padilla, O, Bowen, MA, & Campbell, KS. CD5 signal transduction: positive or negative modulation of antigen receptor signaling. Crit Rev Immunol. (2000). , 20, 347-58.

[51] Raman, C. CD5, an important regulator of lymphocyte selection and immune tolerance. Immunol Res. (2002). , 26, 255-63.

[52] Miller, RA, Oseroff, AR, Stratte, PT, & Levy, R. Monoclonal antibody therapeutic trials in seven patients with T-cell lymphoma. Blood. (1983). , 62, 988-95.

[53] Dillman, RO, Shawler, DL, Dillman, JB, & Royston, I. Therapy of chronic lymphocytic leukemia and cutaneous T-cell lymphoma with T101 monoclonal antibody. J Clin Oncol. (1984). , 2, 881-91.

[54] Ravel, S, Colombatti, M, & Casellas, P. Internalization and intracellular fate of anti-CD5 monoclonal antibody and anti-CD5 ricin A-chain immunotoxin in human leukemic T cells. Blood. (1992). , 79, 1511-7.

[55] Przepiorka, D, Le Maistre, CF, Huh, YO, Luna, M, Saria, EA, Brown, CT, & Champlin, RE. Evaluation of anti-CD5 ricin A chain immunoconjugate for prevention of acute graft-vs.-host disease after HLA-identical marrow transplantation. Ther Immunol. (1994). , 1, 77-82.

[56] Olsen, NJ, Brooks, R. H, Cush, JJ, Lipsky, PE. St Clair, EW, Matteson, EL, Gold, KN, Cannon, GW, Jackson, CG, McCune, WJ, Fox, DA, Nelson, B, Lorenz, T, & Strand, V. A double-blind, placebo-controlled study of anti-CD5 immunoconjugate in patients with rheumatoid arthritis. The Xoma RA Investigator Group. Arthritis Rheum. (1996). , 39, 1102-8.

[57] Ma, A, Koka, R, & Burkett, P. Diverse functions of IL-2, IL-15, and IL-7 in lymphoid homeostasis. Ann Rev Immunol. (2006). , 24, 657-79.

[58] Nelson, BH, & Willerford, DM. Biology of the interleukin-2 receptor. Adv Immunol. (1998). , 70, 1-81.

[59] Waldmann, TA. The structure, function, and expression of interleukin-2 receptors on normal and malignant T-cells. Science. (1986). , 232, 727-32.

[60] Uchiyama, T, Broder, S, & Waldmann, TA. A monoclonal antibody (anti-Tac) reactive with activated and functionally mature human T cells. I. Production of anti-Tac monoclonal antibody and distribution of Tac (+) cells. J Immunol. (1981). , 126, 1393-7.

[61] Queen, C, Schneider, WP, Selick, HE, Payne, PW, Landolfi, NF, Duncan, JF, Avdalovic, NM, Levitt, M, Junghans, RP, & Waldmann, TA. A humanized antibody that binds to the interleukin 2 receptor. Proc Natl Acad Sci USA. (1989). , 86, 10029-33.

[62] Zhang, M, Zhang, Z, Garmestani, K, Goldman, CK, Ravetch, JV, Brechbiel, MW, Carrasquillo, JA, & Waldmann, TA. Activating Fc receptors are required for antitumor efficacy of the antibodies directed toward CD25 in a murine model of adult T-cell leukemia. Cancer Res. (2004). , 64, 5825-9.

[63] Berkowitz, JE, Janik, JE, Stewart, D, Fioravanti, S, Jaffe, ES, Fleisher, TA, Urqhart, N, Wharfe, GH, Waldmann, TA, & Morris, JC. Phase II trial of daclizumab in human T-cell lymphotropic virus type-1 (HTLV-1)-associated adult T-cell leukemia/lymphoma (ATL). J Clin Oncol 28:15s, 2010 (suppl; abstr 8043)

[64] Ansell, SM, Horwitz, SM, Engert, A, Khan, KD, Lin, T, Strair, R, Keler, T, Graziano, R, Blanset, D, Yellin, M, Fischkoff, S, Assad, A, & Borchmann, P. Phase I/II study of an anti-CD30 monoclonal antibody (MDX-060) in Hodgkin's lymphoma and anaplastic large-cell lymphoma. J Clin Oncol. (2007)., 25, 2764-2769.

[65] Younes, A, Gopal, AK, Smith, SE, Ansell, SM, Rosenblatt, JD, Savage, KJ, Ramchandren, R, Bartlett, NL, Cheson, BD, De Vos, S, Forero-torres, A, Moskowitz, CH, Connors, JM, Engert, A, Larsen, EK, Kennedy, DA, Sievers, EL, & Chen, R. Results of a pivotal phase II study of brentuximab vedotin for patients with relapsed or refractory Hodgkin's lymphoma. J Clin Oncol. (2012)., 30, 2183-9.

[66] Pro, B, Advani, R, Brice, P, Bartlett, NL, Rosenblatt, JD, Illidge, T, Matous, J, Ramchandren, R, Fanale, M, Connors, JM, Yang, Y, Sievers, EL, Kennedy, DA, & Shustov, A. Brentuximab vedotin (SGN-35) in patients with relapsed or refractory systemic anaplastic large-cell lymphoma: results of a phase II study. J Clin Oncol. (2012)., 30, 2190-6.

[67] Lozanski, G, Heerema, NA, Flinn, IW, Smith, L, Harbison, J, Webb, J, Moran, M, Lucas, M, Lin, T, Hackbarth, ML, Proffitt, JH, Lucas, D, Grever, MR, & Byrd, JC. (2004). Alemtuzumab is an effective therapy for chronic lymphocytic leukemia with mutations and deletions. Blood. 2004; 103:3278-3281., 53.

[68] Dearden, CE, Matutes, E, Cazin, B, Tjønnfjord, GE, Parreira, A, Nomdedeu, B, Leoni, P, Clark, FJ, Radia, D, Rassam, SM, Roques, T, Ketterer, N, Brito-Babapulle, V, Dyer, MJ, & Catovsky D. High remission rate in T-cell prolymphocytic leukemia with CAMPATH-1H. Blood. (2001)., 98, 1721-1726.

[69] Keating, MJ, Cazin, B, Coutré, S, Birhiray, R, Kovacsovics, T, Langer, W, Leber, B, Maughan, T, Rai, K, Tjønnfjord, G, Bekradda, M, Itzhaki, M, & Hérait P. Campath-1H treatment of T-cell prolymphocytic leukemia in patients for whom at least one prior chemotherapy regimen has failed. J Clin Oncol. (2002)., 20, 205-213.

[70] Lundin, J, Hagberg, H, Repp, R, Cavallin-Ståhl, E, Fredén, S, Juliusson, G, Rosenblad, E, Tjønnfjord, G, Wiklund, T, & Osterborg, A. Phase 2 study of alemtuzumab (anti-CD52 monoclonal antibody) in patients with advanced mycosis fungoides/Sezary syndrome. Blood. (2003)., 101, 4267-4272.

[71] Enblad, G, Hagberg, H, Erlanson, M, Lundin, J, MacDonald, AP, Repp, R, Schetelig, J, Seipelt, G, & Osterborg, A. A pilot study of alemtuzumab (anti-CD52 monoclonal antibody) therapy for patients with relapsed or chemotherapy-refractory peripheral T-cell lymphomas Blood. (2004)., 103, 2920-2924.

[72] Gallamini, A, Zaja, F, Patti, C, Billio, A, Specchia, MR, Tucci, A, Levis, A, Manna, A, Secondo, V, Rigacci, L, Pinto, A, Iannitto, E, Zoli, V, Torchio, P, Pileri, S, & Tarella, C. Alemtuzumab (Campath-1H) and CHOP chemotherapy as first-line treatment of peripheral T-cell lymphoma: results of a GITIL (Gruppo Italiano Terapie Innovative nei Linfomi) prospective multicenter trial. Blood. (2007)., 110, 2316-23.

[73] Kluin-nelemans, HC, van Marwijk Kooy, M, Lugtenburg, PJ, van Putten, WL, Luten, M, Oudejans, J, & van Imhoff, GW. Intensified alemtuzumab-CHOP therapy for peripheral T-cell lymphoma. Ann Oncol. (2011). , 22, 1595-600.

[74] Ravandi, F, Aribi, A, O'Brien, S, Faderl, S, Jones, D, Ferrajoli, A, Huang, X, York, S, Pierce, S, Wierda, W, Kontoyiannis, D, Verstovsek, S, Pro, B, Fayad, L, Keating, M, & Kantarjian, H. Phase II study of alemtuzumab in combination with pentostatin in patients with T-cell neoplasms. J Clin Oncol. (2009). , 27, 5425-5430.

[75] Kobayashi, H, Dubois, S, Sato, N, Sabzevari, H, Sakai, Y, Waldmann, TA, & Tagaya, Y. Role of trans-cellular IL-15 presentation in the activation of NK cell-mediated killing, which leads to enhanced tumor immunosurveillance. Blood. (2005). , 105, 721-7.

[76] Morris, JC, Janik, JE, White, JD, Fleisher, TA, Brown, M, Tsudo, M, Goldman, CK, Bryant, B, Petrus, M, Top, L, Lee, CC, Gao, W, & Waldmann, TA. Preclinical and phase I clinical trial of blockade of IL-15 using Mikbeta1 monoclonal antibody in T cell large granular lymphocyte leukemia. Proc Natl Acad Sci USA. (2006). , 103, 401-6.

[77] Yoshie, O, Fujisawa, R, Nakayama, T, Harasawa, H, Tago, H, Izawa, D, Hieshima, K, Tatsumi, Y, Matsushima, K, Hasegawa, H, Kanamaru, A, Kamihira, S, & Yamada, Y. Frequent expression of CCR4 in adult T-cell leukemia and human T-cell leukemia virus type 1-transformed T cells. Blood. (2002). , 99, 1505-1511.

[78] Ito, A, Ishida, T, Yano, H, Inagaki, A, Suzuki, S, Sato, F, Takino, H, Mori, F, Ri, M, Kusumoto, S, Komatsu, H, Iida, S, Inagaki, H, & Ueda, R. Defucosylated anti-CCR4 monoclonal antibody exercises potent ADCC-mediated antitumor effect in the novel tumor-bearing humanized NOD/Shi-scid, IL-2Rgamma(null) mouse model. Cancer Immunol Immunother. (2009). , 58, 1195-1206.

[79] Yamamoto, K, Utsunomiya, A, Tobinai, K, Tsukasaki, K, Uike, N, Uozumi, K, Yamaguchi, K, Yamada, Y, Hanada, S, Tamura, K, Nakamura, S, Inagaki, H, Ohshima, K, Kiyoi, H, Ishida, T, Matsushima, K, Akinaga, S, Ogura, M, Tomonaga, M, & Ueda, R. Phase I study of KW-0761, a defucosylated humanized anti-CCR4 antibody, in relapsed patients with adult T-cell leukemia-lymphoma and peripheral T-cell lymphoma. J Clin Oncol. (2010). , 28, 1591-1598.

[80] Ishida, T, Joh, T, Uike, N, Yamamoto, K, Utsunomiya, A, Yoshida, S, Saburi, Y, Miyamoto, T, Takemoto, S, Suzushima, H, Tsukasaki, K, Nosaka, K, Fujiwara, H, Ishitsuka, K, Inagaki, H, Ogura, M, Akinaga, S, Tomonaga, M, Tobinai, K, & Ueda, R. Defucosylated anti-CCR4 monoclonal antibody (KW-0761) for relapsed adult T-cell leukemia-lymphoma: a multicenter phase II study. J Clin Oncol. (2012). , 30, 837-42.

Chapter 6

Prevention of Human T-Cell Lymphotropic Virus Infection and Adult T-Cell Leukemia

Makoto Yoshimitsu, Tomohiro Kozako and
Naomichi Arima

Additional information is available at the end of the chapter

1. Introduction

1.1. Prevention of HTLV-1 and adult T cell leukemia/lymphoma (ATLL)

Human T-cell lymphotropic virus type 1 was first discovered as a human retrovirus that causes the T cell hematological malignancy, called adult T cell leukemia/lymphoma[1, 2]. The virus is transmitted through contact with bodily fluids containing HTLV-1 infected cells mostly from mother to child transmission through breastfeeding or blood transfusion. ATLL occur after prolonged incubation periods. Strategies for the prevention of ATLL should be divided into two steps. The first step is the prevention of HTLV-1 transmission. This has been established in some HTLV-1 endemic areas by screening for HTLV-1 among blood donors and refraining from breastfeeding among pregnant women who are HTLV-1 carriers. The second step is the prevention of ATLL development among HTLV-1 carriers. This has not been established at all. Approximately 90% of HTLV-1 carriers remain as healthy as uninfected individuals through their lifetime and the risk factors for developing ATLL remain to be defined. In addition, preventative intervention like vaccination may cause other unfavorable immuno-logical consequences, thus well-examined strategies need to be further developed.

2. Epidemiology of HTLV-1 infection

1.   Worldwide

Nearly 20 million people worldwide are estimated to be infected with HTLV-1[3]. Among them, only less than 10% develop HTLV-1 related disorders including adult T-cell leukemia/

lymphoma throughout their lives. A number of studies regarding the geographical and ethnoepidemiological distribution of the virus have been achieved in last 3 decades [4, 5], and revealed that southwestern Japan, tropical Africa, the Caribbean islands, and Central and South America are the endemic areas in the world. In Europe and North America, the prevalence is limited to the population emigrated from endemic areas.

2. Japan

The result of recent survey revealed that the estimated number of HTLV-1 carriers was at least 1.08 million in Japan[6]. This is 10% lower than that reported in 1988. The estimated prevalence rates were 0.66% in men and 1.02% in women.

3. Mode of transmission

The route of infection has been shown to be related to the development of HTLV-1-associated diseases. ATLL has been mainly associated with breastfeeding and HTLV-1-associated myelopathy/tropical spastic paraparesis has been associated with blood transfusion[7]. ATLL cases of post-transfusion have been scarcely reported[8]. Three major routes of viral transmission have been established: [1] mother-to-child transmission, mainly via breast-feeding[9, 10]; sexual transmission, predominantly male to female[11, 12]; and [3] cellular blood compo-

Prevention of HTLV-1 and ATLL

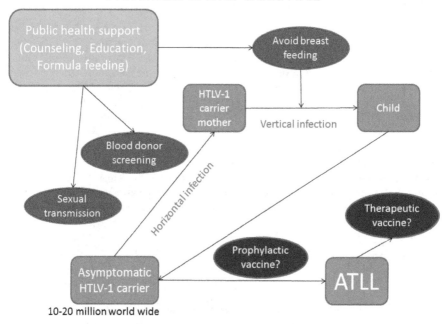

Figure 1. Prevention of HTLV-1 and ATLL

nents[13]. The efficiency of the mother-to-child transmission route is estimated to be around 20%[14]. Mother-to-child transmission during pregnancy or peripartum period has been reported to be less than 5%[15].

3. Epidemiology of adult T cell leukemia/lymphoma

Only a small proportion of HTLV-1 carrier develops ATLL after long latency period. Despite wide geographical distribution, the data regarding the incidence and prevalence of ATLL are scarce except for Japan. In addition the reported data might be underestimated for lymphoma type which resemble to other T cell lymphoma because of the difficulty of definite diagnosis in less developed countries. Among Japanese population, the incidence of ATLL among carriers is estimated to be 4.5-7.3% in men and 2.6-3.5% in women [16-18]. ATLL is reported to develop among individuals predominantly in their fifth decade in Japan [19], in the Jamaican and Brazilian series, patients tend to present the disease in the fourth decade, which suggest other immunological background or local factors may play a role in the disease development[20, 21].

4. Mechanisms of HTLV-1 transmission

HTLV-1 can infect a wide variety of human cell types in vitro [22, 23], thus its receptor is thought to be a ubiquitously expressed molecule. GLUT1, heparin sulfate proteoglycan(HSPG) and neuropilin-1 are the three molecules that are reported as key players for the interaction between the viral envelop and the cell membrane, and for the entry into the cells [24-26]. It has been proposed that HTLV-1 particles first contact HSPG, then neuropilin-1 recruits HTLV-1/ HSPG complex to present them to GLUT1. HSPG/neuropilin-1/GLUT1 complex makes the viral envelop competent for membrane fusion and entry into the cell.

Cell-free HTLV-1 virions are poorly infectious in vitro for most of cell types including their primary target cells, CD4 T cells. The main transmission pattern of HTLV-1 is cell-to-cell contact, however, only myeloid and plasmacytoid dendritic cells can be infected by cell-free HTLV-1[27]. This route may be important in the setting of mother-to-child transmission through breast-feeding. Dendritic cells may play an important role during initial acquisition of infection, milk-to-mucosal transmission of the virus.

Three major mechanisms of cell-to-cell transmission of HTLV-1 have been proposed: [1] HTLV-1-infected lymphocytes polarized their microtubules and viral components upon contact with other T cells, forming so-called virological synapses[28]; [2] HTLV-1-infected cells produce and transiently store viral particles in extracellular adhesive structures rich in extracellular matrix components, including collagen and agrin, and cellular linker proteins, such as tetherin and galectin-3, which resemble bacterial biofilms. Extracellular viral assemblies rapidly adhere to other cells upon cell contact, allowing virus spread and infection of target cells[29]; and [3] HTLV-1–pX region encoded p8 protein increases T-cell conjugation through lymphocyte function-associated antigen-1 clustering. In addition, p8 induces cellular conduits among T cells and increases viral transmission[30].

5. Prevention of transmission of HTLV-1

The prognosis for ATLL is one of the worst among hematological malignancies with best available therapy, and no preventative vaccine against HTLV-1 is yet available. Thus the prevention of transmission of HTLV-1 is the most realistic way to prevent the progression of ATLL.

5.1. Prevention of vertical transmission

Retrospective and prospective epidemiological studies revealed the mother-to-child trans-mission rate was around 20%[14]. Prevention of mother-to-child transmission has the most significant impact on the occurrence of HTLV-1 infection and associated diseases. Avoidance of breastfeeding is of the essence as it is the major form of vertical transmission of this virus. A prefecture-wide intervention study in Nagasaki Prefecture in Southern Japan to refrain from breast-feeding by carrier mothers revealed a marked reduction of HTLV-1 mother-to-child transmission from 20.3% to 2.5%. Thus, prenatal screening for HTLV-1 should be employed in endemic areas, combined with relevant counseling of carrier mothers regarding transmis-sion of HTLV-1 through breastfeeding. Although children breast-fed for less than 6 months has significantly lower incidence of HTLV-1 infection than those breast-fed for more than 6 months, their chances of infection are significantly higher than those of bottle-fed children. Thus exclusive bottle-feeding is recommended[31].

Even with exclusive bottle-feeding, 2.5% of infants born to carrier mothers were infected with HTLV-1. As intrauterine transmission of HTLV-1 should be rare, transplacental transmission during delivery is most likely as is the case for other viruses, i.e. HBV and HCV.

Even though the dramatic impact of bottle feeding on mother-to-child transmission of HTLV-1, public health policies should consider the risk of malnutrition, especially in developing countries where the malnutrition is the primary causes of infant deaths. An alternative feeding formula should be recommended for children at risk of acquiring HTLV-1 infection through mother's milk. The practice of cross-feeding should also be avoided.

5.2. Prevention of horizontal transmission

HTLV-1 can also be spread through contact with bodily fluids such as whole blood or whole blood products. The development of ATLL related to transfusion is exceptional. Thus, the purpose of prevention of horizontal transmission is mainly to reduce HTLV-1 carrier population.

5.3. Transfusion and sexual transmission

HTLV-1 screening program to prevent transfusion-related transmission of HTLV-1 has been developed since 1986 and many countries in endemic areas started to employ systematic screening of all blood donors [7, 32]. Screening of blood donor candidates has been shown to be an effective strategy in preventing HTLV-1 transmission. For HTLV-1 non-endemic areas, reports showed that the risk of HTLV-1 infection might be enhanced in some selected donor populations, especially in immigrants from endemic area, recommending the employment of policies for selective donor recruitment. For developing countries, the high cost of imported screening test kit is not negligible, thus, more cost effective strategies for blood donor screening need to be developed. In most African countries, transfusion still represents a risk of HTLV-1 transmission.

Most of sexual transmission of HTLV-1 is from men to women. Recommendations to prevent sexually transmitted infections should be emphasized, including condom use and avoiding multiple and unknown sexual partners. Nonetheless, access to correct information about HTLV-1 infection and appropriate counseling is very important as blood donor candidates and sexually active people are usually asymptomatic and in reproductive age.

6. Pathogenesis of adult T cell leukemia/lymphoma

The pathogenesis of ATLL is not completely understood. Extensive studies have revealed that HTLV-1 transacting transcriptional activator (Tax) plays a critical role in the transformation of virus infected cells. Tax is thought to be a potent oncoprotein, as it solely immortalizes human primary T cells and Tax transgenic mice develop spontaneous tumors. Tax enhances viral replication through transactivation of the viral promoter, the 5'LTR, and its multifaceted functions including activation of NF-kB pathway, cell cycle progression, induction of aneuploidy, induction of DNA damage and impairment of DNA repair. Thus, Tax is thought to play a key role in the pathogenesis of ATLL[33].

HTLV-1 bZIP factor (HBZ) is encoded in the minus strand of the HTLV-1 provirus, and is ubiquitously expressed in all ATLL cells [34]. HBZ protein was originally reported to suppress Tax-mediated viral transcription, however, HBZ RNA possesses cell proliferation function. Importantly, HBZ transgenic mice developed CD4/Foxp3 positive T-cell lymphoma, which resembles the phenotype of human ATLL. These findings suggest that HBZ is a critical factor in leukemogenesis. Possible hypothesis of the interplay between Tax and HBZ is that Tax is needed to initiate transformation of HTLV-1 infected cells while HBZ is required to maintain the transformed phenotype in ATLL[33].

7. Determinants for ATLL progression inHTLV-1 carriers

The determinants for ATLL progression in HTLV-1 carriers have been investigated in many epidemiological and clinical studies. ATLL is named after its adult onset time of the disease, thus age is the most well-known factor. The recent survey from Japan reported that the age at diagnosis was around 65 years [35]. However the average age at diagnosis of ATLL in Jamaica was mid-forties[36], thus other host factors and environmental characteristics may also affect the disease onset. The age at time of HTLV-1 infection is also a critical factor for ATLL development as ATLL scarcely develops in HTLV-1 carriers by horizontal infection. Early studies suggested that patients with ATLL had more family history of ATLL than that in the general population, thus several host genetic background factors have been investigated including HLA haplotype. The frequency of HLA-A26, HLA-B4002, HLA-B4006 and HLA-B4801 alleles were significantly higher in ATLL patients than in HTLV-1 asymptomatic carriers in Japan [37]. Several laboratory markers were investigated for ATLL development. A series of Miyazaki cohort study reported that HTLV-I carriers with a higher anti-HTLV-I titer and a lower anti-Tax reactivity may be at greatest risk of ATLL [38]. The Miyazaki study also reported that the levels of HTLV-1 proviral load was higher in HTLV-1 carrier who developed ATLL than in asymptomatic HTLV-1 carriers. A nationwide prospective study for HTLV-1 carrier was initiated to investigate the determinant of ATLL development. 14 subjects out of 1218 asymptomatic carrier developed ATLL and all of the 14 subjects had higher baseline proviral load. None developed ATLL among those with a baseline proviral load less than 4 copies/100 peripheral blood mononuclear cells [39].

8. Prognosis of adult T cell leukemia/lymphoma

1.   Acute type and lymphoma type

The prognosis of acute type and lymphoma type of ATLL remain poor with chemotherapy or allogeneic hematopoietic stem cell transplantation. With currently best available chemotherapy [40], the rate of complete response was 40%. Overall survival at 3 years was 24%. The median survival time is 13 months.

2.   Chronic type and smoldering type (indolent type ATLL)

A previous study, in which Japanese patients with ATLL were followed for a maximum duration of 7 years, reported that the 4-year survival rates for chronic, and smoldering type were 26.9%, and 62.8% respectively, with the median survival time (MST) of 24.3 months, and not yet reached, respectively[41].Therefore, the chronic and smoldering subtypes of ATLL are considered indolent and are usually managed with watchful waiting until disease progression to acute crisis, similar to the management of chronic lymphoid leukemia or smoldering myeloma. However, recent report with long term follow-up of indolent ATLL (chronic and smoldering type) revealed that the median survival time was 4.1 years and the estimated 5-, 10-, 15-year survival rates were 47.2%, 25.4% and 14.1%, respectively[42]. The prognosis of indolent ATLL in this study was poorer than expected. These findings suggest that even patients with indolent ATLL should be carefully observed in clinical practice.

9. Current treatment option

9.1. Conventional chemotherapy

The results of a phase III randomized control trial suggest that the vincristine, cyclophosphamide, doxorubicin, and prednisone (VCAP); doxorubicin, ranimustine, and prednisone

(AMP); and vindesine, etoposide, carboplatin, and prednisone (VECP) regimen is not superior to biweekly cyclophosphamide, doxorubicin, vincristine, and prednisone (CHOP) in newly diagnosed acute, lymphoma, or unfavorable chronic types of ATLL in terms of overall survival(OS), which is primary endpoint of this study, or progression free survival [40].However, the rate of complete response (CR) was higher in the VCAP-AMP-VECP arm than the biweekly CHOP arm [40% v 25%, respectively; $P=0.020$). OS at 3 years was 24% in the VCAP-AMP-VECP arm and 13% in the CHOP arm ($P= 0.085$). Nonetheless, the median survival time of 13 months still compares unfavorably to other hematologic malignancies.

9.2. Allogeneic hematopoietic stem cell transplantation (alloHSCT)

alloHSCT has been explored as promising alternative therapeutic modality that can provide long-term remission in a proportion of patients with ATLL[43-45]. In a recent large nationwide retrospective analysis, investigators compared outcomes of 386 patients with ATL who underwent allogeneic HSCT. After a median follow-up of 41 months, 3-year overall survival for entire cohort was 33% [45]. Retrospective analysis based on 294 ATLL patients who received alloHSCT revealed that the development of mild-to-moderate acute GVHD confers a lower risk of disease progression and a beneficial influence on survival [46], which is the indicative of the presence of a graft-versus-ATLL effect. Another large retrospective analysis of alloHSCT for ATLL (n=586) in Japan revealed that no significant difference in OS between myeloablative conditioning (MAC) and reduced intensity conditioning (RIC) regimen was observed. There was a trend indicating that RIC contributed to better OS in older patients[47]. The number of ATLL patients eligible for allogeneic transplantation is quite limited because of older age at presentation and the low rate of CR. Selection criteria of alloHSCT for patients with ATLL remain to be determined.

9.3. Interferon-α (IFN-α) and zidovudine (AZT)

The results of a recent worldwide meta-analysis on the use of AZT/IFN for 254 ATLL patients, the treatment of ATLL patients with AZT and IFN resulted in better response and prolonged overall survival[48]. Two hundred seven patients received first-line AZT/IFN therapy. In these patients, five-year overall survival rates were 46% for 75 patients who received first-line antiviral therapy (P = 0.004). In acute ATLL, achievement of complete remission with antiviral therapy resulted in 82% 5-year survival. These results suggest that treatment of ATLL using AZT/IFN results in high response and CR rates except for lymphoma type of ATLL, resulting in prolonged survival in a significant proportion of patients. Although this is a retrospective analysis, the results seem to be promising, and further studies comparing AZT/IFN-α and conventional chemotherapy or alloHSCT are warranted.

10. Prevention of ATLL

The prevention of ATLL mostly relies on the prevention of HTLV-1 transmission as previously described. Another way is the prevention of ATLL development among HTLV-1 carriers. Even though long-term opportunity to intervene the HTLV-1 carrier status, this has not been achieved at all at any stages. This is partly because only approximately 10% of HTLV-1 carriers develop HTLV-1 related disease in their lifetime. Risk-benefit balance including acceptable side effect during intervention are needed to be carefully assessed.

11. Future direction of prevention of ATLL development

11.1. Immunological impairment of HTLV-1 specific T cells

Vertical transmission, high proviral loads, and suppression of HTLV-1-specific T-cell immune responses are reported to be associated with risk factors for ATLL development. It has been reported that Tax specific cytotoxic T lymphocytes (CTLs) detected in chronic and smoldering ATLL and subset of asymptomatic carriers are anergic to antigen stimulation [49]. Such functional impairment of CTLs seems specific to HTLV-1 as cytomegalovirus-specific CTLs remain intact.

In animal models, oral inoculation of HTLV-1 virions induces T cell tolerance against HTLV-1[50]. As breast feeding is the main route of vertical transmission in HTLV-1 infection, this may induce neonatal T cell tolerance against HTLV-1.

In addition to immunological tolerance, T cell exhaustion may be another mechanism of antigen-specific T cell suppression. We have reported PD-1 expression on Tax-specific CTLs may indicate Tax-specific T cell exhaustion [51].

12. Vaccine

Vaccination of HTLV-1 against uninfected individuals is not sophisticated strategy for prevention of ATLL as most of ATLL develop after long incubation period among vertically transmitted HTLV-1 carriers within 6 months of their lives and vertical transmissions are almost completely prevented by refraining breastfeeding. Thus, the purpose of vaccination is to augment HTLV-1-specific T-cell response to reduce the risk of development of ATLL in such above mentioned subpopulation.

i.   HTLV-1 Tax-targeted vaccines in a rat model of HTLV-1-induced lymphomas showed promising antitumor effects [52]. In addition, the HTLV-1-immunized monkeys developed a strong cellular immune response with HTLV-1 specific-peptides and a significant reduction in the proviral load was observed in these immunized monkeys after challenge [53]. Therefore, these results provide a rationale for clinical use of such a vaccine for preventing ATLL. However, there are several obstacles to overcome for clinical use. One major obstacle is that HTLV-1 specific synthetic peptides are poorly immunogenic to elicit efficient induction of antigen-specific CTLs. We have explored the efficient induction of HTLV-1-specific T cell responses by oligomannose-coated liposomes (OMLs) encapsulating the HLA-

A*0201-restricted HTLV-1 Tax-epitope (OML/Tax)[54]. Immunization of HLA-A*0201 transgenic mice with OML/Tax resulted in the efficient induction of HTLV-1-specific IFN-γ producing T cells. Dendritic cells (DCs) exposed to OML/Tax showed increased expression of DC maturation markers. In addition, HTLV-1-Tax-specific CD8+ T cells were efficiently induced by OML/Tax derived from HTLV-1 carriers. OML/Tax increased the number of HTLV-1-specific CD8+ T cells by average 170-fold, while treatment without antigen showed an increase of 9-fold. Furthermore, these HTLV-1-specific CD8+ cells efficiently lysed HTLV-1 epitope peptide-pulsed T2-A2 cells. These results suggest that OML/Tax induces antigen-specific cellular immune responses without the need for adjuvants and may be an effective vaccine carrier to augment HTLV-1-specific T-cell response to reduce the risk of development of ATLL.

ii.   Nonetheless, for the clinical use of HTLV-1 vaccine, extraction of high risk group for ATLL needs to be clearly defined to avoid unwanted immunological consequence including other HTLV-1 associated inflammatory diseases.

13. Conclusion

So far, the prevention of ATLL totally relies on the prevention of vertical HTLV-1 transmission by refraining breastfeeding from HTLV-1 carrier mother. Prenatal screening of HTLV-1 should be implemented in the endemic area with careful counseling. In addition, screening of blood donor candidates has been shown to be effective in preventing HTLV-1 transmission. Recommendations to prevent sexual-transmission should be emphasized, including condom use and adopting safe sexual behavior. The development of an effective and safe vaccine should be emphasized.

Author details

Makoto Yoshimitsu[1*], Tomohiro Kozako[2] and Naomichi Arima[1,3]

*Address all correspondence to: myoshimi@m.kufm.kagoshima-u.ac.jp

1 Department of Hematology and Immunology, Kagoshima University Hospital, Kagoshima, Japan

2 Department of Biochemistry, Faculty of Pharmaceutical Sciences, Fukuoka University, Fukuoka, Japan

3 Division of Hematology and Immunology, Center for chronic viral diseases, Graduate School of Medical and Dental Sciences, Kagoshima, Japan

References

[1] Poiesz, B. J, Ruscetti, F. W, Gazdar, A. F, Bunn, P. A, Minna, J. D, & Gallo, R. C. Detection and isolation of type C retrovirus particles from fresh and cultured lymphocytes of a patient with cutaneous T-cell lymphoma. Proc Natl Acad Sci U S A. (1980). Dec;, 77(12), 7415-9.

[2] Yoshida, M, Miyoshi, I, & Hinuma, Y. Isolation and characterization of retrovirus from cell lines of human adult T-cell leukemia and its implication in the disease. Proc Natl Acad Sci U S A. (1982). Mar;, 79(6), 2031-5.

[3] De The, G, & Kazanji, M. An HTLV-I/II vaccine: from animal models to clinical trials? J Acquir Immune Defic Syndr Hum Retrovirol. (1996). Suppl 1:S, 191-8.

[4] Goncalves, D. U, Proietti, F. A, Ribas, J. G, Araujo, M. G, Pinheiro, S. R, Guedes, A. C, et al. Epidemiology, treatment, and prevention of human T-cell leukemia virus type 1-associated diseases. Clin Microbiol Rev. (2010). Jul;, 23(3), 577-89.

[5] Sonoda, S, Li, H. C, & Tajima, K. Ethnoepidemiology of HTLV-1 related diseases: ethnic determinants of HTLV-1 susceptibility and its worldwide dispersal. Cancer Sci. (2011). Feb;, 102(2), 295-301.

[6] Satake, M, Yamaguchi, K, & Tadokoro, K. Current prevalence of HTLV-1 in Japan as determined by screening of blood donors. J Med Virol. (2012). Feb;, 84(2), 327-35.

[7] Osame, M, Janssen, R, Kubota, H, Nishitani, H, Igata, A, Nagataki, S, et al. Nationwide survey of HTLV-I-associated myelopathy in Japan: association with blood transfusion. Ann Neurol. (1990). Jul;, 28(1), 50-6.

[8] Chen, Y. C, Wang, C. H, Su, I. J, Hu, C. Y, Chou, M. J, Lee, T. H, et al. Infection of human T-cell leukemia virus type I and development of human T-cell leukemia lymphoma in patients with hematologic neoplasms: a possible linkage to blood transfusion. Blood. (1989). Jul;, 74(1), 388-94.

[9] Yamanouchi, K, Kinoshita, K, Moriuchi, R, Katamine, S, Amagasaki, T, Ikeda, S, et al. Oral transmission of human T-cell leukemia virus type-I into a common marmoset (Callithrix jacchus) as an experimental model for milk-borne transmission. Jpn J Cancer Res. (1985). Jun;, 76(6), 481-7.

[10] Kinoshita, K, Amagasaki, T, Hino, S, Doi, H, Yamanouchi, K, Ban, N, et al. Milk-borne transmission of HTLV-I from carrier mothers to their children. Jpn J Cancer Res. (1987). Jul;, 78(7), 674-80.

[11] Tajima, K, Tominaga, S, Suchi, T, Kawagoe, T, Komoda, H, Hinuma, Y, et al. Epidemiological analysis of the distribution of antibody to adult T-cell leukemia-virus-associated antigen: possible horizontal transmission of adult T-cell leukemia virus. Gann. (1982). Dec;, 73(6), 893-901.

[12] Murphy, E. L, Figueroa, J. P, Gibbs, W. N, Brathwaite, A, Holding-cobham, M, Waters, D, et al. Sexual transmission of human T-lymphotropic virus type I (HTLV-I). Ann Intern Med. (1989). Oct 1;, 111(7), 555-60.

[13] Okochi, K, & Sato, H. Transmission of ATLV (HTLV-I) through blood transfusion. Princess Takamatsu Symp. (1984). , 15, 129-35.

[14] Hino, S, Yamaguchi, K, Katamine, S, Sugiyama, H, Amagasaki, T, Kinoshita, K, et al. Mother-to-child transmission of human T-cell leukemia virus type-I. Jpn J Cancer Res. (1985). Jun;, 76(6), 474-80.

[15] Fujino, T, & Nagata, Y. HTLV-I transmission from mother to child. J Reprod Immunol. (2000). Jul;, 47(2), 197-206.

[16] Tokudome, S, Tokunaga, O, Shimamoto, Y, Miyamoto, Y, Sumida, I, Kikuchi, M, et al. Incidence of adult T-cell leukemia/lymphoma among human T-lymphotropic virus type I carriers in Saga, Japan. Cancer Res. (1989). Jan 1;, 49(1), 226-8.

[17] Koga, Y, Iwanaga, M, Soda, M, Inokuchi, N, Sasaki, D, Hasegawa, H, et al. Trends in HTLV-1 prevalence and incidence of adult T-cell leukemia/lymphoma in Nagasaki, Japan. J Med Virol. (2010). Apr;, 82(4), 668-74.

[18] Kondo, T, Kono, H, Miyamoto, N, Yoshida, R, Toki, H, Matsumoto, I, et al. Age- and sex-specific cumulative rate and risk of ATLL for HTLV-I carriers. Int J Cancer. (1989). Jun 15;, 43(6), 1061-4.

[19] Takatsuki, K, Matsuoka, M, & Yamaguchi, K. Adult T-cell leukemia in Japan. J Acquir Immune Defic Syndr Hum Retrovirol. (1996). Suppl 1:S, 15-9.

[20] Gibbs, W. N, Lofters, W. S, Campbell, M, & Hanchard, B. LaGrenade L, Cranston B, et al. Non-Hodgkin lymphoma in Jamaica and its relation to adult T-cell leukemia-lymphoma. Ann Intern Med. (1987). Mar;, 106(3), 361-8.

[21] Pombo de Oliveira MS, Matutes E, Schulz T, Carvalho SM, Noronha H, Reaves JD, et al. T-cell malignancies in Brazil. Clinico-pathological and molecular studies of HTLV-I-positive and-negative cases. Int J Cancer. (1995). Mar 16;, 60(6), 823-7.

[22] Sommerfelt, M. A, Williams, B. P, Clapham, P. R, Solomon, E, Goodfellow, P. N, & Weiss, R. A. Human T cell leukemia viruses use a receptor determined by human chromosome 17. Science. (1988). Dec 16;, 242(4885), 1557-9.

[23] Koyanagi, Y, Itoyama, Y, Nakamura, N, Takatsu, K, Kira, J, Iwamasa, T, et al. In vivo infection of human T-cell leukemia virus type I in non-T cells. Virology. (1993). Sep;, 196(1), 25-33.

[24] Manel, N, Kim, F. J, Kinet, S, Taylor, N, Sitbon, M, & Battini, J. L. The ubiquitous glucose transporter GLUT-1 is a receptor for HTLV. Cell. (2003). Nov 14;, 115(4), 449-59.

[25] Jones, K. S, Petrow-sadowski, C, Bertolette, D. C, Huang, Y, & Ruscetti, F. W. Heparan sulfate proteoglycans mediate attachment and entry of human T-cell leukemia virus type 1 virions into CD4+ T cells. J Virol. (2005). Oct;, 79(20), 12692-702.

[26] Lambert, S, Bouttier, M, Vassy, R, Seigneuret, M, Petrow-sadowski, C, Janvier, S, et al. HTLV-1 uses HSPG and neuropilin-1 for entry by molecular mimicry of VEGF165. Blood. (2009). May 21;, 113(21), 5176-85.

[27] Jones, K. S, Petrow-sadowski, C, Huang, Y. K, Bertolette, D. C, & Ruscetti, F. W. Cell-free HTLV-1 infects dendritic cells leading to transmission and transformation of CD4(+) T cells. Nat Med. (2008). Apr;, 14(4), 429-36.

[28] Igakura, T, Stinchcombe, J. C, Goon, P. K, Taylor, G. P, Weber, J. N, Griffiths, G. M, et al. Spread of HTLV-I between lymphocytes by virus-induced polarization of the cytoskeleton. Science. (2003). Mar 14;, 299(5613), 1713-6.

[29] Pais-correia, A. M, Sachse, M, Guadagnini, S, Robbiati, V, Lasserre, R, Gessain, A, et al. Biofilm-like extracellular viral assemblies mediate HTLV-1 cell-to-cell transmission at virological synapses. Nat Med. (2010). Jan;, 16(1), 83-9.

[30] Van Prooyen, N, Gold, H, Andresen, V, Schwartz, O, Jones, K, Ruscetti, F, et al. Human T-cell leukemia virus type 1 protein increases cellular conduits and virus transmission. Proc Natl Acad Sci U S A. (2010). Nov 30;107(48):20738-43., 8.

[31] Hino, S. Establishment of the milk-borne transmission as a key factor for the peculiar endemicity of human T-lymphotropic virus type 1 (HTLV-1): the ATL Prevention Program Nagasaki. Proc Jpn Acad Ser B Phys Biol Sci. (2011). , 87(4), 152-66.

[32] Inaba, S, Sato, H, Okochi, K, Fukada, K, Takakura, F, Tokunaga, K, et al. Prevention of transmission of human T-lymphotropic virus type 1 (HTLV-1) through transfusion, by donor screening with antibody to the virus. One-year experience. Transfusion. (1989). Jan;, 29(1), 7-11.

[33] Matsuoka, M, & Jeang, K. T. Human T-cell leukemia virus type 1 (HTLV-1) and leukemic transformation: viral infectivity, Tax, HBZ and therapy. Oncogene. (2011). Mar 24;, 30(12), 1379-89.

[34] Satou, Y, Yasunaga, J, Yoshida, M, & Matsuoka, M. HTLV-I basic leucine zipper factor gene mRNA supports proliferation of adult T cell leukemia cells. Proc Natl Acad Sci U S A. (2006). Jan 17;, 103(3), 720-5.

[35] Yamada, Y, Atogami, S, Hasegawa, H, Kamihira, S, Soda, M, Satake, M, et al. Nationwide survey of adult T-cell leukemia/lymphoma (ATL) in Japan. Rinsho Ketsueki. (2011). Nov;, 52(11), 1765-71.

[36] Hanchard, B. Adult T-cell leukemia/lymphoma in Jamaica: J Acquir Immune Defic Syndr Hum Retrovirol. (1996). Suppl 1:S20-5., 1986-1995.

[37] Yashiki, S, Fujiyoshi, T, Arima, N, Osame, M, Yoshinaga, M, Nagata, Y, et al. HLA-A*26, HLA-B*4002, HLA-B*4006, and HLA-B*4801 alleles predispose to adult T cell

leukemia: the limited recognition of HTLV type 1 tax peptide anchor motifs and epitopes to generate anti-HTLV type 1 tax CD8(+) cytotoxic T lymphocytes. AIDS Res Hum Retroviruses. (2001). Jul 20;, 17(11), 1047-61.

[38] Hisada, M, Okayama, A, Shioiri, S, Spiegelman, D. L, Stuver, S. O, & Mueller, N. E. Risk factors for adult T-cell leukemia among carriers of human T-lymphotropic virus type I. Blood. (1998). Nov 15;, 92(10), 3557-61.

[39] Iwanaga, M, Watanabe, T, Utsunomiya, A, Okayama, A, Uchimaru, K, Koh, K. R, et al. Human T-cell leukemia virus type I (HTLV-1) proviral load and disease progression in asymptomatic HTLV-1 carriers: a nationwide prospective study in Japan. Blood. (2010). Aug 26;, 116(8), 1211-9.

[40] Tsukasaki, K, Utsunomiya, A, Fukuda, H, Shibata, T, Fukushima, T, Takatsuka, Y, et al. VCAP-AMP-VECP compared with biweekly CHOP for adult T-cell leukemia-lymphoma: Japan Clinical Oncology Group Study JCOG9801. J Clin Oncol. (2007). Dec 1;, 25(34), 5458-64.

[41] Shimoyama, M. Diagnostic criteria and classification of clinical subtypes of adult T-cell leukaemia-lymphoma. A report from the Lymphoma Study Group (1984-87). Br J Haematol. (1991). Nov;, 79(3), 428-37.

[42] Takasaki, Y, Iwanaga, M, Imaizumi, Y, Tawara, M, Joh, T, Kohno, T, et al. Long-term study of indolent adult T-cell leukemia-lymphoma. Blood. (2010). Jun 3;, 115(22), 4337-43.

[43] Utsunomiya, A, Miyazaki, Y, Takatsuka, Y, Hanada, S, Uozumi, K, Yashiki, S, et al. Improved outcome of adult T cell leukemia/lymphoma with allogeneic hematopoietic stem cell transplantation. Bone Marrow Transplant. (2001). Jan;, 27(1), 15-20.

[44] Choi, I, Tanosaki, R, Uike, N, Utsunomiya, A, Tomonaga, M, Harada, M, et al. Long-term outcomes after hematopoietic SCT for adult T-cell leukemia/lymphoma: results of prospective trials. Bone Marrow Transplant. (2011). Jan;, 46(1), 116-8.

[45] Hishizawa, M, Kanda, J, Utsunomiya, A, Taniguchi, S, Eto, T, Moriuchi, Y, et al. Transplantation of allogeneic hematopoietic stem cells for adult T-cell leukemia: a nationwide retrospective study. Blood. (2010). Aug 26;, 116(8), 1369-76.

[46] Kanda, J, Hishizawa, M, Utsunomiya, A, Taniguchi, S, Eto, T, Moriuchi, Y, et al. Impact of graft-versus-host disease on outcomes after allogeneic hematopoietic cell transplantation for adult T-cell leukemia: a retrospective cohort study. Blood. (2012). Mar 1;, 119(9), 2141-8.

[47] Ishida, T, Hishizawa, M, Kato, K, Tanosaki, R, Fukuda, T, Taniguchi, S, et al. Allogeneic hematopoietic stem cell transplantation for adult T-cell leukemia-lymphoma with special emphasis on preconditioning regimen: a nationwide retrospective study. Blood. (2012). Aug 23;, 120(8), 1734-41.

[48] Bazarbachi, A, & Plumelle, Y. Carlos Ramos J, Tortevoye P, Otrock Z, Taylor G, et al. Meta-analysis on the use of zidovudine and interferon-alfa in adult T-cell leukemia/

lymphoma showing improved survival in the leukemic subtypes. J Clin Oncol. (2010). Sep 20;, 28(27), 4177-83.

[49] Takamori, A, Hasegawa, A, Utsunomiya, A, Maeda, Y, Yamano, Y, Masuda, M, et al. Functional impairment of Tax-specific but not cytomegalovirus-specific CD8+ T lymphocytes in a minor population of asymptomatic human T-cell leukemia virus type carriers. Retrovirology. (2011)., 1.

[50] Hasegawa, A, Ohashi, T, Hanabuchi, S, Kato, H, Takemura, F, Masuda, T, et al. Expansion of human T-cell leukemia virus type 1 (HTLV-1) reservoir in orally infected rats: inverse correlation with HTLV-1-specific cellular immune response. J Virol. (2003). Mar;, 77(5), 2956-63.

[51] Kozako, T, Yoshimitsu, M, Fujiwara, H, Masamoto, I, Horai, S, White, Y, et al. PD-1/PD-L1 expression in human T-cell leukemia virus type 1 carriers and adult T-cell leukemia/lymphoma patients. Leukemia. (2009). Feb;, 23(2), 375-82.

[52] Ohashi, T, Hanabuchi, S, Kato, H, Tateno, H, Takemura, F, Tsukahara, T, et al. Prevention of adult T-cell leukemia-like lymphoproliferative disease in rats by adoptively transferred T cells from a donor immunized with human T-cell leukemia virus type 1 Tax-coding DNA vaccine. J Virol. (2000). Oct;, 74(20), 9610-6.

[53] Kazanji, M, Heraud, J. M, Merien, F, Pique, C, De The, G, Gessain, A, et al. Chimeric peptide vaccine composed of B- and T-cell epitopes of human T-cell leukemia virus type 1 induces humoral and cellular immune responses and reduces the proviral load in immunized squirrel monkeys (Saimiri sciureus). J Gen Virol. (2006). May; 87(Pt 5):1331-7.

[54] Kozako, T, Hirata, S, Shimizu, Y, Satoh, Y, Yoshimitsu, M, White, Y, et al. Oligomannose-coated liposomes efficiently induce human T-cell leukemia virus-1-specific cytotoxic T lymphocytes without adjuvant. FEBS J. (2011). Apr;, 278(8), 1358-66.

Chapter 7

The Roles of AMP-Activated Protein Kinase-Related Kinase 5 as a Novel Therapeutic Target of Human T-Cell Leukaemia Virus Type 1-Infected T-Cells

Mariko Tomita

Additional information is available at the end of the chapter

1. Introduction

HTLV-1 (human T-cell leukemia virus type 1) is a human retrovirus and the causative agent of ATL (adult T-cell leukemia), which is an aggressive and fatal T cell malignancy characterized by dysregulated proliferation of CD4-positive T cells [1-3]. HTLV-1 causes ATL in 3-5% of infected individuals after a long latent period of 40-60 years [4]. The prognosis of patients with aggressive ATL remains poor with a median survival time of less than 1 year despite advances in both chemotherapy and supportive care [5, 6]. Infiltration of leukemic cells into various organs, such as lymph nodes, liver, spleen, lung, skin and intestinal tract, is a frequent manifestation of ATL. This type of cell infiltration often poses serious clinical problems for ATL patients, affecting the disease profile and prognosis. Because tumor cell survival and growth are maintained by nutrients, especially glucose and oxygen supplied by blood vessels, angiogenesis is considered to be essential for tumor malignancy [7].

Currently, the molecular mechanism of malignant transformation by HTLV-1 remains undefined. However, Tax, the 40-kDa transactivator protein encoded by HTLV-1, plays a crucial role in T cell transformation and leukemogenesis. Tax triggers viral transcription as well as induction of cellular genes involved in cell proliferation and anti-apoptotic signaling. In addition to activation of transcription, Tax transforms the infected cells by some mechanisms due to protein-protein interaction between Tax and other proteins [8, 9]. Moreover, one key feature of ATL is aneuploidy and chromosomal instability. Tax also contributes transformation of the cells by inducing aneuploidy and inactivating chromosomal instability checkpoint [10]. Indeed, it immortalizes primary human T cells derived from peripheral blood or cord blood [11, 12] and induces tumors and leukemia in transgenic mice [13, 14].

NF-κB (nuclear factor κB) is a major survival signaling pathway activated by HTLV-1. This pathway is constitutively active in HTLV-1-transformed T-cells and primary ATL cells [15, 16].Tax can activate NF-κB pathway by associating with various signaling molecules in this pathway. For example, Tax binds IKKγ (also known as NEMO) and triggers the phosphorylation of IKKα and IKKβ, which form a complex with IKKγ [15]. Subsequently the IKK complex phosphorylates IκBα, leading to its proteasome-mediated degradation, which frees IκBα-sequestered cytoplasmic NF-κB to migrate into the nucleus where it activates the transcription of NF-κB-responsive genes [15]. Tax can also stimulate an alternative NF-κB pathway through the IKKα-dependent processing of the NF-κB p100 precursor protein to its active p52 form [17]. The NF-κB signaling pathways are activated in ATL cells that do not express Tax, although the mechanism of activation remains unknown [16]. One of the potential mechanisms by which ATL cells could develop resistance to apoptosis is through the activation of NF-κB. From this point of view, NF-κB has become an attractive target for therapeutic intervention.

AMPK (AMP-activated protein kinases) are a class of serine/threonine kinases that are activated by increased intracellular concentrations of AMP. ARK5 is a fifth member of the AMPK catalytic subunit family [18-20], and involved in tumor invasion and metastasis [21], and also known to induce cell survival during nutrient starvation or death receptor activation [22, 23]. ARK5 promoter contains two putative MARE (Maf-recognition element) sequences [24]. The *maf* proto-oncogene is identified within the genome of the avian musculoaponeurotic fibrosarcoma virus, AS42 [25]. The products of the Maf family share a conserved bZip motif that mediates dimer formation and DNA binding to the MARE [26]. Transcription of *ARK5* gene is regulated by the large Maf-family proteins including c-Maf and MafB. ARK5 is induced when a c-Maf or MafB expression vector is introduced into non-ARK5-expressing colon cancer cells [24]. Deregulated expression of ARK5 is also associated with Maf-transforming activity in human angioimmunoblastic T-cell lymphoma and in Maf-driven T-cell lymphoma in transgenic mice [27]. In multiple myeloma cells, over expression of ARK5 correlates with the expression of c-Maf and MafB and exhibits increased invasiveness [24]. ARK5 mRNA expression in colon cancer is stage-associated and liver metastatic foci of colon cancer express very high levels of ARK5 mRNA [28, 29]. In this study, we focused on ARK5 and analyzed its expression and role on the growth of HTLV-1-infected T-cells.

2. Materials and methods

2.1. Reagents

Bay 11-7082 and LY294002 were purchased from Calbiochem. D-(+)-glucose was purchased from Nakalaitesque.

2.2. Cell lines

The HTLV-1-uninfected T-cell leukemia cell lines MOLT-4 and CCRF-CEM, the HTLV-1-infected T-cell lines MT-2 [30], MT-4 [31],C5/MJ [32], SLB-1 [33], HUT-102 [1], MT-1 [34] and TL-OmI [35]were maintained in RPMI 1640 medium supplemented with 10% heat-inactivated fetal bovine serum, 50 units/ml penicillin, and 50 μg/ml streptomycin (Sigma-Aldrich) at

$37°C$ in 5% CO_2. MT-2, MT-4, C5/MJ and SLB-1 are HTLV-1-transformed T-cell lines which were established by an *in vitro* coculture protocol. MT-1 and TL-OmI are leukemic T-cell lines derived from patients with ATL. HUT-102 was established from a patient with ATL, but its clonal origin is unclear. TY8-3 is an IL-2-dependent cell line established from a thymoma specimen of a myasthenia gravis patient. TY8-3/MT-2 cells were established from TY8-3 cells by coculture with mitomycin C-treated HTLV-1-infected MT-2 cells in the presence of IL-2 [36]. JPX-9 and JPX/M (kindly provided by Dr. M. Nakamura, Tokyo Medical and Dental University, Tokyo, Japan) are subclones of Jurkat cells that express Tax wild type and Tax mutant protein defective in its some abilities including activation of NF-κB, respectively, under the control of the metallothionein promoter [37]. Expression of Tax was induced by addition of $CdCl_2$ to a final concentration of 20 μM.

2.3. RT (reverse transcriptase)-PCR

Total cellular RNA was extracted from cells using Trizol reagent as described by the supplier (Invitrogen). First-strand cDNA was synthesized in a 10-μl reaction volume using RNA-PCR kit (TAKARA BIO) with random primers. Thereafter, cDNA was amplified for ARK5 and c-Maf. The oligonucleotide primers used were as follows: for ARK5; sense, 5'- GAGTCCACTC-TATGCATC-3' and antisense, 5'- ATGTCCTCAATAGTGGCC-3'; for c-Maf; sense, 5'-TGCACTTCGACGACCGCTTCT C-3' and antisense, 5'- CGCTGCTCGAGCCGTTTTCTC-3'. Product sizes were 256-bp for ARK5 and 327-bp for c-Maf. The amplification programs were follows: denaturing at $94°C$ for 2 min, an annealing step at $55°C$ for 30 s and an extension step at $72°C$ for 30 s. Amplification cycles were 35 cycles for ARK5 and c-Maf, 25 cycles for β-actin. The PCR products were fractionated on 2% agarose gels and visualized by ethidium bromide staining.

2.4. Real-time RT-PCR

Total RNA was extracted from cells with Trizol reagent. Total RNA was reverse transcribed to obtain single-strand cDNA with High Capacity cDNA Reverse Transcription Kit (Applied Biosystems). PCR was carried out in a total volume of 25 μl of reaction mixture containing 1 μl of diluted cDNA, 12.5 μl of Brilliant SYBR® Green QPCR Master Mix (Stratagene), and 100 nM of each primer with a Mx3000P® Real-Time PCR System (Stratagene). For precise quantitative determination of the transcripts, we assessed the expression levels of GAPDH as an internal control. PCR conditions were set according to the instructions supplied by the manufacturer. The real-time PCR assay of each sample was conducted in triplicate, and the mean value was used as the mRNA level. The PCR primer pairs used in this study for ARK5 and c-Maf are listed above and those for Tax and GAPDH were as follow: for Tax; sense, 5'-CCCACTTCCCAGGGTTTGGACAGA-3' and antisense, 5'- CTGTAGAGCTGAGCCGA-TAACGCG-3'; for GAPDH; sense, 5'-GAGTCAACGGATTTGGTCGT-3' and antisense, 5'-GACAAGCTTCCCGTTCTCAG-3'.

2.5. Western blot analysis

Western blot analysis was performed as described previously [38]. In brief, cells were lysed in sodium dodecyl sulfate (SDS) sample buffer containing 62.5 mM Tris-HCl (pH 6.8), 2% (wt/vol) SDS, 10% glycerol, 6% 2-mercaptoethanol and 0.01% bromophenol blue. The lysates were resolved by electrophoresis on polyacrylamide gels and then electroblotted onto poly-vinylidene difluoride membranes (Millipore). The membranes were incubated overnight with the appropriate primary antibody, as indicated, at 4°C. After washing, the blots were exposed to the appropriate secondary antibody conjugated with horseradish peroxidase for 1 h at room temperature. The reaction products were visualized using enhanced chemilumi-nescence reagent (GE Healthcare) according to the instructions provided by the manufactur-er. We used primary antibodies against Tax (Lt-4) [39], phosphorylated IκBα (Ser32/36), phosphorylated AKT(Ser473), AKT, NF-κB (p65) (Cell Signaling Technology), IκBα, (Santa Cruz Biotechnology) and actin (Lab Vision). Horseradish-peroxidase-conjugated secondary antibodies were purchased from GE Healthcare.

2.6. Plasmids

The reporter assay construct for ARK5 promoter was described previously [24]. In brief, based on the results of a Genomic BLAST Search, primers with the NheI (upstream primer) or XhoI (downstream primer) site were synthesized, and PCR was then performed with the primers for genomic DNA extracted from PANC-1 cells. The PCR fragment digested with NheI and XhoI was ligated into pGL2-basic.A series of expression vectors for Tax (Tax WT) and mutants thereof (Tax M22 and Tax 703) were described previously [40, 41]. IκBα ΔN and IκBβ ΔN are deletion mutants of IκBα and IκBβ lacking the N-terminal 36 amino acids and 23 amino acids, respectively. IKKβ K44A and NEMOΔC are the dominant negative mu-tants of IKKβ and NEMO, respectively [42, 43]. The expression vector for mouse c-Maf was described previously [44]. NF-κB (p65) expression plasmid was described previously [45].

2.7. Transfection and luciferase assay

Transfections were performed in CCRF-CEM cells by electroporation with Microporator MP-100® (Digital Bio Technology) according to the instructions supplied by the manufactur-er for optimization and use. In all cases, the reference plasmid phRL-TK, which contains the *Renilla* luciferase gene under the control of the Herpes simplex virus thymidine kinase pro-moter, was cotransfected to correct for transfection efficiency. Then cells were collected by centrifugation and lysed in reporter lysis buffer (Promega). Luciferase assays were per-formed by using the Dual-Luciferase Reporter System (Promega), in which relative lucifer-ase activities were calculated by normalizing transfection efficiency according to the *Renilla* luciferase activities.

2.8. siRNA (small interfering RNA)

To knockdown ARK5 and c-Maf expression, predesigned double-stranded siRNAs (siGE-NOME SMART pool Human ARK5 and Human MAF;Dharmacon) were used. The siCON-

TROL non-targeting siRNA pool (Dharmacon) was used as a negative control. siRNAs were transfected into MT-2 cells by electroporation with MicroporatorMP-100®.

2.9. EMSA (electrophoretic mobility-shift assay)

Nuclear extracts were prepared from cells and DNA-binding activity was analyzed by EMSA, as described previously [16]. Briefly, 5 µg of nuclear extracts were pre-incubated in a binding buffer containing 1 µg poly-deoxy-inosinic-deoxy-cytidylic acid (Amersham Biosciences), followed by addition of [α-^{32}P]-labeled oligonucleotide probe. These mixtures were incubated for 15 min at room temperature. The DNA-protein complexes were separated on 4% polyacrylamide gels and visualized by autoradiography. The probes or competitors used were prepared by annealing the following sense and antisense synthetic oligonucleotides: NF-κB binding sites ARK5 κB A and ARK5 κB B derived from the ARK5 gene promoter 5′- gatcCTCTTGGGGTTCTCCTGGAC-3′ and 5′-gatcAGGTGGGG-GAAGCCCTGGCT-3′, respectively. Mutants ARK5 κB A and ARK5 κB B are 5′-gatcCTCTTGGCCACGAGCTGGAC-3′and 5′-gatcAGGTGGGCCTCCAGCTGGCT-3′, respectively. To identify NF-κB proteins in the DNA-protein complex identified by EMSA, we used antibodies specific for various NF-κB family proteins, including p50, p65, c-Rel, RelB and p52 (Santa Cruz Biotechnology), to elicit a supershift DNA-protein complex formation. These antibodies were incubated with the nuclear extracts for 45 min at room temperature before incubation with radiolabeled probes.

2.10. Cell proliferation assay

The cells transfected with siRNA were incubated for 12 h, then seeded into 24-well plates at 1×10^5 viable cells per well, and incubated in glucose-containing or non-containing medium for the indicated time periods. The number of viable cells was determined every 24 h by counting trypan blue-excluding cells in a hemocytometer.

2.11. Statistical analysis

Data were expressed as mean ± SD. Differences between groups were analyzed by the unpaired Student's t-test. A p value less than 0.05 denoted the presence of a statistically significant difference.

3. Results

3.1. ARK5 and c-Maf are highly expressed in HTLV-1-infected T-cell lines

Expression of ARK5 and c-Maf mRNA was examined in 6 HTLV-1-infected (MT-2, MT-4, C5/MJ, SLB-1, HUT-102, MT-1 and TL-OmI) and 2 HTLV-1-uninfected (MOLT-4 and CCRF-CEM) T-cell lines. ARK5 mRNAs were detectable in all HTLV-1-infected T-cell lines, but not in uninfected T-cell lines (Figure 1A, left panel). c-Maf expression was relatively higher in HTLV-1-infected T-cell lines than in HTLV-1-uninfected T-cell lines (Figure 1A, right panel).

The high expression of MafB was detected only in HTLV-1-infected MT-2 cells, but no differences in expression were noted between other infected and uninfected T-cell lines (results not shown). Although Tax protein was not detectable in ATL-derived T-cell lines (Figure 1C), Tax mRNA was expressed in all HTLV-1-infected T-cell lines by real time RT-PCR, which is more sensitive method than Western blot (Figure 1B). These results suggest a close association between HTLV-1 infection and induction of ARK5 and c-Maf mRNA expression.

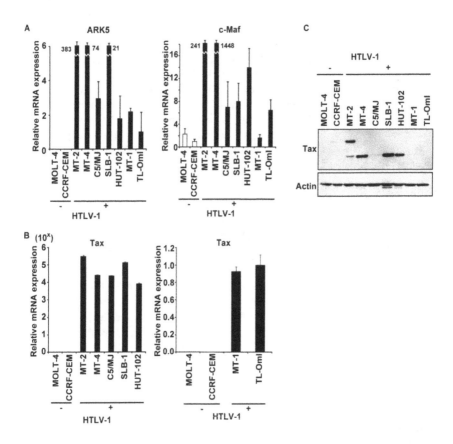

Figure 1. Overexpression of ARK5 and c-Maf in HTLV-1-infected T-cell lines. The expressions of ARK5, c-Maf (A) and Tax (B) mRNAs were analyzed in HTLV-1-infected (HTLV-1; +) and uninfected (HTLV-1; -) T-cell lines by real time RT-PCR. Results are shown as fold change of mRNA expression relative to that of TL-Oml (ARK5 and Tax) or CCRF-CEM (c-Maf). Real time RT-PCR data were obtained using the ΔΔCt method, with normalization to the reference GAPDH mRNA. Data are mean ± SD of triplicate experiments. Numbers on MT-2, MT-4, and SLB-1 represent the actual values. (C) Western blotting was used to determine the expression of Tax protein. Actin was a loading control.

3.2. HTLV-1 Tax induces ARK5 and c-Maf expression in T cells

To examine the direct association between ARK5 or c-Maf mRNAs induction and HTLV-1 infection, we used HTLV-1-infected TY8-3/MT-2 cells, which were established from TY8-3 cells by cocultivation with HTLV-1-infected MT-2 cells [36]. Although MafB expression level was slightly increased in TY8-3/MT-2 cells (results not shown), the expression of ARK5 and c-Maf mRNAs was clearly higher in TY8-3/MT-2 cells than parental TY8-3 cells (Figure 2A). Because Tax induces various cellular genes, we next examined whether this includes the expression of ARK5 and c-Maf mRNAs in T cells. We used JPX-9 cells, which stably carry Tax expression plasmid, in which Tax expression is induced by the addition of $CdCl_2$ [37]. The expression of ARK5, c-Maf, and Tax mRNAs was analyzed by real time RT-PCR (Figure 2B). The addition of $CdCl_2$ to the culture medium of JPX-9 cells induced the expression of Tax within 2 h, which persisted until 72 h after treatment. A concomitant increase of ARK5 mRNA within 10 h of treatment with $CdCl_2$ was observed in JPX-9 cells. Rapid expression of c-Maf mRNA was also observed within 2 h, and peaked after 10 h of treatment with $CdCl_2$. The induction of ARK5 or c-Maf could not be attributed to $CdCl_2$ treatment, since ARK5 or c-Maf expression was not induced in JPX/M cells, which express Tax mutant protein, after treatment with $CdCl_2$ (results not shown). These results indicate that Tax can increase the expression of ARK5 and c-Maf in T cells.

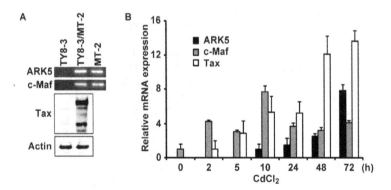

Figure 2. HTLV-1 Tax induces the expression of ARK5 and c-Maf mRNAs. (A) Infection of HTLV-1 induced ARK5 and c-Maf mRNA expression. The expression levels of ARK5 and c-Maf mRNAs in TY8-3 cells and HTLV-1-infected TY8-3 cells established by coculture with MT-2 cells were analyzed by RT-PCR. MT-2 was a positive control. Representative results of three experiments with similar results. (B) Tax expression was induced by adding $CdCl_2$ (20 μM) in JPX-9 cells. Cells were harvested at the indicated time points. ARK5, c-Maf, and Tax mRNA expression levels were analyzed by real time RT-PCR. Results are shown as fold change of mRNA expression relative to that at 0 h (c-Maf), 2 h (Tax), and 10 h (ARK5). Real time RT-PCR data were obtained using the $\Delta\Delta$Ct method, with normalization to the reference GAPDH mRNA. Data are mean ± SD of triplicate experiments.

3.3. c-Maf does not alter ARK5 expression in T cells

ARK5 gene promoter contains two putative MARE sequences [24]. c-Maf and MafB induce the gene transcription through interaction with MARE on the promoter region of target gene [26, 46]. ARK5 is induced when a c-Maf expression vector is introduced into non-ARK5-expressing colon cancer cells [24]. Our findings of a strong correlation between ARK5 and c-Maf expression in HTLV-1-infected T-cell lines and Tax inducible JPX-9 cells suggest that ARK5 could be regulated by c-Maf which is induced by Tax in these cells. However, transient transfection of c-Maf expression plasmid into ARK5-negative CCRF-CEM cells did not induce ARK5 mRNA expression (Figure 3A). Furthermore, c-Maf did not induce transcriptional activation of *ARK5* gene promoter reporter plasmid (Figure 3B) and knockdown of c-Maf expression in MT-2 cells by siRNA did not affect the expression level of ARK5 mRNA (Figure 3C). These results suggest that c-Maf does not contribute to induction of ARK5 transcription in T lymphocytes.

3.4. Tax activates ARK5 transcriptional activity through NF-κB pathway

Next, we investigated whether Tax could directly enhance the activity of *ARK5* promoter. CCRF-CEM cells were transiently transfected with a reporter gene construct containing the *ARK5* promoter together with Tax. Tax enhanced the transcriptional activity of this reporter (Figure 4A). We analyzed the nucleotide database and found two putative NF-κB sites on the promoter of *ARK5* gene. Tax stimulates transcription through distinct transcription factors, such as NF-κB and CREB (cyclic AMP response element-binding protein). Therefore, we tested two mutant forms of Tax; Tax M22 and Tax 703 [40, 41], to investigate whether Tax-mediated activation of NF-κB signaling pathway was required for induction of the *ARK5* promoter activation in T cells. Tax M22 activates CREB but does not affect NF-κB, while Tax 703 activates NF-κB but does not affect CREB [41]. In the present experiments, Tax 703, but not Tax M22, activated the *ARK5* promoter reporter (Figure 4A). Blocking NF-κB signaling pathway using various dominant negative forms of these signaling molecules reduced Tax-induced activation of *ARK5* promoter (Figure 4B). The nuclear extracts from HTLV-1-infected T-cell lines showed high NF-κB DNA-binding activity by EMSA using both NF-κB binding sites; denoted as ARK5 κB A and B sites, in the *ARK5* promoter as probes. In contrast, no significant DNA-binding activity was detected in extracts of HTLV-1-uninfected T-cell lines (Figure 4C). Competition and supershift assays showed that the observed DNA-protein complexes were specific for either ARK5 κB A or B site and included NF-κB components; p50, p65 or c-Rel proteins (Figure 4D). Transient transfection of NF-κB p65 expression plasmid in CCRF-CEM cells showed that overexpression of NF-κB p65 induced promoter activity of *ARK5* gene (Figure 4E) and expression of ARK5 mRNA (Figure 4F). These results suggest that NF-κB activation directly contributes to induction of the *ARK5* gene expression by Tax.

3.5. NF-κB inhibitor suppresses ARK5 expression in an HTLV-1-infected T-cell line

NF-κB is constitutively activated not only in HTLV-1 transformed T-cell lines but also in ATL-derived T-cell lines and primary ATL cells [16]. We analyzed the effects of an NF-κB inhibitor Bay11-7082, an inhibitor of phosphorylation of IκBα, on the expression of ARK5 in an HTLV-1-infected T-cell line. The expression of ARK5 mRNA in MT-2 cells was reduced by treatment with Bay11-7082 (Figure 5A, left panels). Inhibition of phosphorylation of IκBα and stabilization of IκBα protein were confirmed by Western blotting (Figure 5A, upper right panels). LY249002, a PI3K (phosphatidyl inositol3-kinase)/AKT inhibitor, did not affect the expression of ARK5 (Figure 5A, left panels). Using Western blotting, we also confirmed inhibition of phosphorylation of AKT by LY294002 (Figure 5A, lower right panels). Inhibition of NF-κB DNA-binding activity by Bay11-7082 was also detected by EMSA using oligonucleotide probes of ARK5 κB A and B sites (Figure 5B). These results support out findings in Figure 4 that indicate the contribution of NF-κB signaling to induction of *ARK5* gene expression in HTLV-1-infected T-cells.

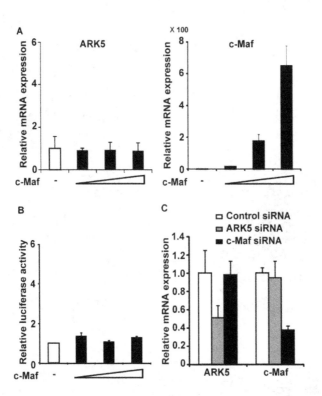

Figure 3. Maf does not affect ARK5 expression in T-cells. (A) c-Maf does not induce ARK5 mRNA expression in HTLV-1-negative T cells. ARK5 mRNA expression in CCRF-CEM cells 48 h after transfection with increasing amounts of c-Maf expression plasmids (0, 0.1, 0.5 and 1 μg) were analyzed by real time RT-PCR (left panel). Transfected c-Maf mRNA expression was confirmed by real time RT-PCR (right panel). (B) c-Maf does not induce *ARK5* promoter activity. CCRF-CEM cells were transfected with increasing amount of c-Maf expression plasmid together with *ARK5*promoter reporter plasmid. Cells were harvested 48 h after transfection and luciferase activity was analyzed. Data are mean ± SD of triplicate experiments. (C) Knockdown of c-Maf did not reduce ARK5 expression in HTLV-1-infected T cells. MT-2 cells were transfected with either ARK5, c-Maf or control siRNA (100nM). The expressions of c-Maf and ARK5 mRNAs were analyzed by RT-PCR. β-actin was a loading control. Representative results of triplicate experiments with similar results.

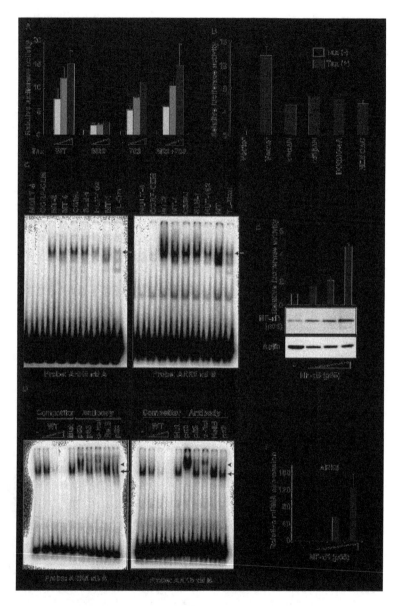

Figure 4. Tax activates ARK5 promoter activity via NF-κB signaling pathway. (A) CCRF-CEM cells were transfected with increasing amounts (0, 0.1, 0.5or 1 μg) of Tax wild type (WT) or mutant (M22 and 703: deficient in NF-κB and CREB signaling activation, respectively) expression plasmids together with ARK5 gene promoter reporter plasmid. Cells were collected 48 hr after transfection and luciferase activity was analyzed. Data are mean ± SD of triplicate experiments. The activity was expressed relative to that of cells transfected with reporter plasmid alone, which was defined as 1. (B)

CCRF-CEM cells were transfected with various dominant negative forms of NF-κB signaling proteins (0.1 μg) and Tax expression plasmid (1 μg) together with ARK5 reporter plasmid. Cells were harvested 48 h after transfection and luciferase activity was analyzed. Data are mean ± SD of triplicate experiments. The activity was expressed relative to that of cells transfected with reporter plasmid alone, which was defined as 1. (C) DNA-binding of NF-κB proteins to ARK5 gene promoter in HTLV-1-infected T-cell lines. DNA-binding of NF-κB proteins to ARK5 promoter was analyzed by EMSA using the ARK5 κB A (top) andARK5 κB B (bottom) oligonucleotide probes containing the NF-κB-binding sites from ARK5 gene. (D) NF-κB subunit specificity was determined using nuclear extracts from MT-2 cells and antibodies to NF-κB components p50, p65, c-Rel, RelB and p52, resulting in super shift. Cold competition using 1, 10 or 100-fold excess of unlabeled probes (wild type probe; WT) or 100-fold excess mutated probe(mutant probe; Mut) demonstrated the specificity of the protein-DNA-binding complex. Arrows indicate specific complexes of NF-κB with ARK5 κB A or ARK5 κB B oligonucleotides, and arrowheads indicate super shift of the bands by antibodies against p50, p65, or c-Rel. (E) NF-κB p65 activates ARK5 promoter activity. CCRF-CEM cells were transfected with increasing amounts (0, 0.1, 0.5 or 1 μg) of NF-κB p65 expression plasmid together with ARK5 promoter reporter plasmid. Cells were harvested 48 h after transfection and luciferase activity was analyzed. Data are mean ± SD of triplicate experiments. The activity was expressed relative to that of cells transfected with reporter plasmid alone, which was defined as 1. The expression of NF-κB p65 was confirmed by Western blotting (lower panel). (F) The expression of ARK5 mRNA induced by NF-κB p65 was analyzed by real time RT-PCR.

3.6. ARK5 maintains tolerance to glucose starvation in HTLV-1-infected T-cells

Finally, we investigated the role of ARK5 on the growth of HTLV-1-infected T-cells. Knockdown of ARK5 expression in MT-2 (Figure 6A, upper panels) and HUT-102 (Figure 6A, lower panels) cells did not affect growth of cells in the complete medium, which contained 2000 mg/mL glucose (Figure 6A, left panels). In contrast, knockdown of ARK5 expression reduced the cell growth in the glucose-free medium (Figure 6A, right panels). The knockdown efficiency was analyzed by real-time RT-PCR and almost equal knockdown efficiency was detected between with and without glucose conditions in both cell lines (Figure 6B). These results suggest that ARK5 maintains tolerance to glucose starvation in HTLV-1-infected T-cells.

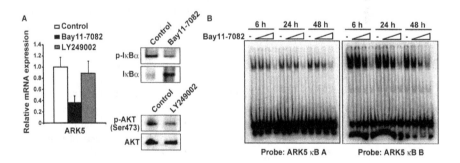

Figure 5. NF-κB inhibitor suppresses ARK5 expression in an HTLV-1-infected T-cell line. (A) MT-2 cells were treated with IκBα phosphorylation inhibitor Bay11-7082 (10 μM) or PI3K inhibitor LY249002 (20 μM) for 24 h. ARK5 expression was analyzed by real time RT-PCR (left panel). Inhibition of phosphorylation and stabilization of IκBα protein by treatment with Bay11-7082 and inhibition of phosphorylation of AKT by treatment with LY249002 were confirmed by Western blotting (right panels). (B) NF-κB inhibitor reduces DNA-binding of NF-κB protein to ARK5 gene promoter in an HTLV-1-infected T-cell line. MT-2 cells were treated with increasing amounts of Bay 11-7082 (0, 1, 5 or 10 μM) for the indicated time periods. DNA-binding of NF-κB proteins to ARK5 promoter was analyzed by EMSA using the ARK5 κB A (top) andARK5 κB B(bottom) oligonucleotide probes containing the NF-κB-binding sites from ARK5 gene.

4. Discussion

Some tumor cells have a strong tolerance to nutrient starvation; tolerance to glucose starvation can be induced by hypoxia. AKT and AMPK appear to be involved closely in the mechanism of tolerance [47-49]. ATL cells often invade the lung, liver, bone, intestine and nerves. Invading leukemia cells might be under nutrient-starvation condition. Therefore, we investigated the roles of ARK5, which is a member of the AMPK family and downstream target of AKT in leukemogenesis by HTLV-1. The results of this study showed high expression of ARK5 and c-Maf in HTLV-1-infected T-cells and that such expression was induced by HTLV-1 Tax (Figure 1 and 2). The promoter region of ARK5 gene has MARE site where c-Maf binds and activates transcription [24]. Unexpectedly, c-Maf induced neither transcriptional activity of ARK5 promoter nor expression of ARK5 mRNA in T lymphocytes (Figure 3), suggesting that transactivation of ARK5 promoter through MARE by c-Maf is cell type-dependent. What is the important transcription factor that inducesARK5 gene expression? We analyzed the nucleotide database and found two putative NF-κB sites on the promoter of ARK5 gene. Tax induced the transcriptional activity of ARK5 gene promoter through activation of NF-κB signaling pathway (Figure 4). This is the first report showing the involvement of NF-κB in the transcription of ARK5 gene.

NF-κB signaling pathway is not only activated by Tax but also constitutively activated in primary ATL cells which express little amount of Tax [16]. Therefore, NF-κB inhibitors are promising therapeutic agents for ATL. At present, several trials are being conducted using the Bay11-7082 [50] and the proteasome inhibitor PS-341 [51] for treatment of ATL. Recently, a new NF-κB inhibitor, dehydroxy-methyle poxy-quinomicin, has been found to inhibit NF-κB signaling pathway induced by Tax as well as the constitutive NF-κB activation in primary ATL cells, without affecting normal peripheral blood mononuclear cells [52, 53]. In the present study, we demonstrated that Bay11-7082 reduced ARK5 expression in an HTLV-1-infected T-cell line (Figure 5), suggesting that NF-κB inhibitors may modulate ATL cells invasion into multiple organs.

Another important finding in this study is that ARK5 is necessary for the growth of HTLV-1-infected T-cells during glucose starvation (Figure 6). Previously, we and others have demonstrated activation of PI3K/AKT signaling in HTLV-1-infected T-cells and Tax-expressing cells [54]. These findings are important because PI3K/AKT signaling is required for malignant growth of HTLV-1-infected T-cells [55, 56]. However, there are numerous other downstream targets of PI3K/AKT [57]. ARK5, one of the downstream targets of PI3K/AKT signaling, contains the consensus sequence of the AKT phosphorylation at amino acids 595-600, and is directly activated by AKT [21, 23]. We propose that Tax has dual roles as an accelerator to induce glucose tolerance in HTLV-1-infected T-cells (Figure 7); 1) induction of ARK5 expression through NF-κB activation (present study), and 2) activation of PI3K/AKT signaling pathway [55, 56].

The molecular mechanisms of induction of tolerance to glucose starvation by ARK5 in HTLV-1-infected T-cells are not elucidated in this study. Previous studies showed that during glucose starvation, survival of human hepatoma HepG2 cells is induced by ARK5 and activation of ARK5 by AKT is necessary for this effect [22, 23]. Glucose tolerance induced by ARK5 in HTLV-1-infected T-cells may also require phosphorylation and activation of ARK5 by AKT. However, we did not analyze the phosphorylation levels or activity of ARK5 in HTLV-1-infected T-cell lines, because a suitable antibody that can recognize phosphorylated ARK5 is not available commercially at present time. ARK5 also negatively regulates death receptors, such as Fas ligand-, TNF-and TRAIL-mediated cell death [22, 58]. When Fas is activated by the ligation of Fas ligand, intracellular interaction of the Fas-death domain, FADD and caspase-8 (death-inducing signaling complex (DISC) recruitment) is initiated for the activation of executioner caspase [59], and c-FLIP is the inhibitor of DISC recruitment. ARK5 directly inactivates caspase-6 through the phosphorylation at Ser^{257}, resulting in c-FLIP preservation, which in turn suppresses DISC formation [58]. Although cell death during glucose starvation is independent of death receptor, DISC recruitment is needed to induce cell death [22]. In this way, ARK5 may prevent cell death during glucose starvation.

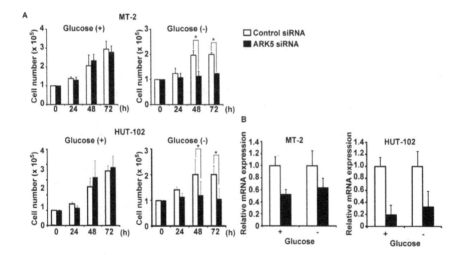

Figure 6. ARK5 maintains tolerance to glucose starvation in HTLV-1-infected T-cell lines. (A) MT-2 cells were transfected with either ARK5 siRNA (solid bars) or control siRNA (open bars) at final concentration of 100 nM. Cells were incubated in glucose containing (+; 2000 mg/L) or glucose-free (-) RPMI for the indicated time points. The effect of siRNA on cell growth was examined by counting the number of viable cells in triplicate by trypanblue dye-exclusion method. Data are mean ± SD of triplicate experiments (*p<0.05). (B) Efficacy of knockdown by ARK5 siRNA in either glucose-containing or glucose-free medium was determined by detecting the expression of ARK5 mRNA by real-time RT-PCR. Results are shown as fold change of mRNA expression relative to that in control siRNA transfected cells. Real-time RT-PCR data were obtained using the ΔΔCt method, with normalization to the reference GAPDH mRNA. Data are mean ± SD of triplicate experiments.

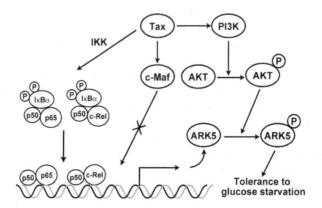

Figure 7. Schematic representation of the effects of Tax on ARK5 expression and AKT activation. Tax induces ARK5 expression by activating NF-κB signaling pathway. AKT is phosphorylated and activated through Tax-induced activation of PI3K. c-Maf is also induced by Tax, but it does not induce ARK5 expression. Activated AKT could phosphorylate and activate ARK5, resulting in tolerance to glucose starvation.

The results showed that c-Maf is highly expressed in HTLV-1-infected T-cells and induced by Tax in T cells (Figure 1 and 2). A previous study showed that c-Maf is expressed in ATL cells in lymph nodes of patients [27]. c-Maf transgenic mice develop T-cell lymphoma and ARK5 is upregulated in c-Maf transgenic thymocytes and T lymphoma cells [27]. In contrast, we found that c-Maf did not activate ARK5 promoter transcription in T-cells. However, c-Maf encodes a Th2-specific transcription factor that activates the expression of IL-4 and IL-10 in T cells [60]. In this regard, a subpopulation of ATL cells produces Th2-associated cytokines [61]. Taken together, it is of interest to identify other downstream target genes responsible for the actions of c-Maf that might contribute to malignant transformation of T cells. For example, some of the target genes of c-Maf, such as those that encode cyclin D2 and integrin β7, have deregulated expression in c-Maf transgenic mice [27]. It might be interesting to investigate the role of c-Maf in the regulation of expression of these genes in ATL cells.

5. Conclusion

We demonstrated overexpression of ARK5 in HTLV-1-infected T-cells and that Tax induced *ARK5* expression by activating the NF-κB signaling pathway. The results also indicated that ARK5 enhanced the growth of HTLV-1-infected T-cells during glucose starvation. The PI3K/AKT pathway, because of its central roles in cell survival, is a target for induction of cell death in HTLV-1-infected T-cells. Thus, ARK5, a downstream target of this pathway, becomes an attractive target in treatment of ATL with invasion of leukemia cells into multiple tissues.

Acknowledgements

We thank the Fujisaki Cell Center, Hayashibara Biomedical Laboratories (Okayama, Japan) for providing HUT-102 cell line, M. Nakamura for providing JPX-9 and JPX/M cells, K. Matsumoto for providing Tax WT, Tax M22 and Tax 703, D.W. Ballard for providing the dominant-negative IκBα and IκBβ (IκBαΔN and IκBβΔN), K.-T. Jeang for providing the dominant-negative NEMO (NEMOΔC) and R. Geleziunas for providing the dominant-negative IKKβ (IKKβK44A) plasmid. We also thank Drs. Kohei Taniguchi, Atsushi Suzuki, Tetsuro Nakazato, Taeko Okudaira, Chie Ishikawa, Yuetsu Tanaka, Satoru Takahashi, Hiroyasu Esumi and Naoki Mori for providing materials, useful comments and discussions. We also acknowledge all members of our laboratories for the helpful comments and collaborations.

This work was supported in part by grants-in-aid for Scientific Research on Priority Areas from the Ministry of Education, Culture, Sports, Science and Technology of Japan, Scientific Research (C) from Japan Society for the Promotion of Science.

No potential conflicts of interest were disclosed.

Abbreviations

ATL, adult T-cell leukemia;

AMPK, AMP-activated protein kinases;

ARK5, AMP-activated protein kinase-related kinase 5;

CREB, cyclic AMP response element-binding protein;

DISC, death-inducing signaling complex;

HTLV-1, human T-cell leukemia virus type 1;

EMSA, electrophoretic mobility-shift assay;

MARE, Maf-recognition element;

NF-κB, nuclear factor-kappa B;

PI3K, phosphatidyl inositol 3-kinase;

RT, reverse transcriptase;

SDS, sodium dodecyl sulfate;

siRNA, small interfering RNA;

WT, wild type.

Author details

Mariko Tomita*

Address all correspondence to: mtomita@med.u-ryukyu.ac.jp

Department of Pathology & Oncology, Graduate School of Medical Science, University of the Ryukyus, Nishihara, Okinawa, Japan

References

[1] Poiesz BJ., Ruscetti FW., Gazdar AF., Bunn PA., Minna JD., Gallo RC. Detection and isolation of type C retrovirus particles from fresh and cultured lymphocytes of a patient with cutaneous T-cell lymphoma. Proceedings of the National Academy of Sciences of the United States of America 1980; 77(12) 7415-7419.

[2] Hinuma Y., Nagata K., Hanaoka M., Nakai M., Matsumoto T., Kinoshita KI., Shirakawa S., Miyoshi I. Adult T-cell leukemia: antigen in an ATL cell line and detection of antibodies to the antigen in human sera. Proceedings of the National Academy of Sciences of the United States of America 1981; 78(10) 6476-6480.

[3] Yoshida M., Miyoshi I., Hinuma Y. Isolation and characterization of retrovirus from cell lines of human adult T-cell leukemia and its implication in the disease. Proceedings of the National Academy of Sciences of the United States of America 1982; 79(6) 2031-2035.

[4] Tajima K. The 4th nation-wide study of adult T-cell leukemia/lymphoma (ATL) in Japan: estimates of risk of ATL and its geographical and clinical features. The T- and B-cell Malignancy Study Group. International Journal of Cancer 1990; 45(2) 237-243.

[5] Yamada Y., Tomonaga M., Fukuda H., Hanada S., Utsunomiya A., Tara M., Sano M., Ikeda S., Takatsuki K., Kozuru M., Araki K., Kawano F., Niimi M., Tobinai K., Hotta T., Shimoyama M. A new G-CSF-supported combination chemotherapy, LSG15, for adult T-cell leukaemia-lymphoma: Japan Clinical Oncology Group Study 9303. British Journal of Haematology 2001; 113(2) 375-382.

[6] Siegel RS.,Gartenhaus RB., Kuzel TM. Human T-cell lymphotropic-I-associated leukemia/lymphoma. Current Treatment Options in Oncology 2001; 2(4) 291-300.

[7] Folkman J. Can mosaic tumor vessels facilitate molecular diagnosis of cancer? Proceedings of the National Academy of Sciences of the United States of America 2001; 98(2) 398-400.

[8] Boxus M., Twizere JC., Legros S., Dewulf JF., Kettmann R., Willems L. The HTLV-1 Tax interactome.Retrovirology 2008; 5 76.

[9] Ramadan E., Ward M., Guo X., Durkin SS., Sawyer A., Vilela M., Osgood C., Pothen A., Semmes OJ. Physical and in silico approaches identify DNA-PK in a Tax DNA-damage response interactome.Retrovirology 2008; 5 92.

[10] Matsuoka M., Jeang KT. Human T-cell leukaemia virus type 1 (HTLV-1) infectivity and cellular transformation. Nature Reviews Cancer 2007; 7(4) 270-280.

[11] Grassmann R., Dengler C., Muller-Fleckenstein I., Fleckenstein B., McGuire K., Dokhelar MC., Sodroski JG., Haseltine WA. Transformation to continuous growth of primary human T lymphocytes by human T-cell leukemia virus type I X-region genes transduced by a Herpesvirussaimiri vector. Proceedings of the National Academy of Sciences of the United States of America 1989; 86(9) 3351-3355.

[12] Grassmann R., Berchtold S., Radant I., Alt M., Fleckenstein B., Sodroski JG., Haseltine WA., Ramstedt U. Role of human T-cell leukemia virus type 1 X region proteins in immortalization of primary human lymphocytes in culture. Journal of Virology 1992; 66(7) 4570-4575.

[13] Nerenberg M., Hinrichs SH., Reynolds RK.,Khoury G., Jay G. The tat gene of human T-lymphotropic virus type 1 induces mesenchymal tumors in transgenic mice. Science 1987; 237(4820) 1324-1329.

[14] Hasegawa H., Sawa H., Lewis MJ., Orba Y., Sheehy N., Yamamoto Y., Ichinohe T., Tsunetsugu-Yokota Y., Katano H., Takahashi H., Matsuda J., Sata T., Kurata T., Nagashima K., Hall WW. Thymus-derived leukemia-lymphoma in mice transgenic for the Tax gene of human T-lymphotropic virus type I. Nature Medicine 2006; 12(4) 466-472.

[15] Sun SC., Yamaoka S. Activation of NF-κB by HTLV-I and implications for cell transformation. Oncogene 2005; 24(39) 5952-5964.

[16] Mori N., Fujii M., Ikeda S., Yamada Y., Tomonaga M., Ballard DW., Yamamoto N. Constitutive activation of NF-κB in primary adult T-cell leukemia cells. Blood 1999; 93(7) 2360-2368.

[17] Xiao G., Cvijic ME., Fong A., Harhaj EW., Uhlik MT., Waterfield M., Sun SC. Retroviral oncoprotein Tax induces processing of NF-κB2/p100 in T cells: evidence for the involvement of IKKα. EMBO Journal 2001; 20(23) 6805-6815.

[18] HardieDG., Carling D. The AMP-activated protein kinase--fuel gauge of the mammalian cell? European Journal of Biochemistry 1997; 246(2) 259-273.

[19] Kemp BE., Stapleton D., Campbell DJ., Chen ZP., Murthy S., Walter M., Gupta A., Adams JJ., Katsis F., van Denderen B., Jennings IG., Iseli T., Michell BJ., Witters LA. AMP-activated protein kinase, super metabolic regulator. Biochemical Society Transactions 2003; 31(Pt 1) 162-168.

[20] Kemp BE., Mitchelhill KI., Stapleton D., Michell BJ., Chen ZP., Witters LA. Dealing with energy demand: the AMP-activated protein kinase. Trends in Biochemical Sciences 1999; 24(1) 22-25.

[21] Suzuki A., Lu J., Kusakai G., Kishimoto A., Ogura T., Esumi H. ARK5 is a tumor in-
      vasion-associated factor downstream of Akt signaling. Molecular and Cellular Biolo-
      gy 2004; 24(8) 3526-3535.

[22] Suzuki A., Kusakai G., Kishimoto A., Lu J., Ogura T., Esumi H. ARK5 suppresses the
      cell death induced by nutrient starvation and death receptors via inhibition of cas-
      pase 8 activation, but not by chemotherapeutic agents or UV irradiation. Oncogene
      2003; 22(40) 6177-6182.

[23] Suzuki A., Kusakai G., Kishimoto A., Lu J., Ogura T., Lavin MF., Esumi H. Identifica-
      tion of a novel protein kinase mediating Akt survival signaling to the ATM protein.
      Journal of Biological Chemistry 2003; 278(1) 48-53.

[24] Suzuki A., Iida S., Kato-Uranishi M., Tajima E., Zhan F., Hanamura I., Huang Y.,
      Ogura T., Takahashi S., Ueda R., Barlogie B., Shaughnessy J, Jr.., Esumi H. ARK5 is
      transcriptionally regulated by the Large-MAF family and mediates IGF-1-induced
      cell invasion in multiple myeloma: ARK5 as a new molecular determinant of malig-
      nant multiple myeloma. Oncogene 2005; 24(46) 6936-6944.

[25] Nishizawa M., Kataoka K., Goto N., Fujiwara KT., Kawai S. v-maf, a viral oncogene
      that encodes a "leucine zipper" motif. Proceedings of the National Academy of Scien-
      ces of the United States of America 1989; 86(20) 7711-7715.

[26] Kataoka K., Noda M., Nishizawa M. Maf nuclear oncoprotein recognizes sequences
      related to an AP-1 site and forms heterodimers with both Fos and Jun. Molecular and
      Cellular Biology 1994; 14(1) 700-712.

[27] Morito N., Yoh K., Fujioka Y., Nakano T., Shimohata H., Hashimoto Y., Yamada A.,
      Maeda A., Matsuno F., Hata H., Suzuki A., Imagawa S., Mitsuya H., Esumi H., Koya-
      ma A., Yamamoto M., Mori N., Takahashi S. Overexpression of c-Maf contributes to
      T-cell lymphoma in both mice and human. Cancer Research 2006; 66(2) 812-819.

[28] Kusakai G., Suzuki A., Ogura T., Miyamoto S., Ochiai A., Kaminishi M., Esumi H.
      ARK5 expression in colorectal cancer and its implications for tumor progression. The
      American journal of pathology 2004; 164(3) 987-995.

[29] Kusakai G., Suzuki A., Ogura T., Kaminishi M., Esumi H. Strong association of ARK5
      with tumor invasion and metastasis. Journal of Experimental & Clinical Cancer Re-
      search 2004; 23(2) 263-268.

[30] Miyoshi I., Kubonishi I., Yoshimoto S., Akagi T., Ohtsuki Y., Shiraishi Y., Nagata K.,
      Hinuma Y. Type C virus particles in a cord T-cell line derived by co-cultivating nor-
      mal human cord leukocytes and human leukaemic T cells. Nature 1981; 294(5843)
      770-771.

[31] Yamamoto N., Okada M., Koyanagi Y., Kannagi M., Hinuma Y. Transformation of
      human leukocytes by cocultivation with an adult T cell leukemia virus producer cell
      line. Science 1982; 217(4561) 737-739.

[32] Popovic M., Sarin PS., Robert-Gurroff M., Kalyanaraman VS., Mann D., Minowada J.,
      Gallo RC. Isolation and transmission of human retrovirus (human t-cell leukemia vi-
      rus). Science 1983; 219(4586) 856-859.

[33] KoefflerHP., Chen IS., Golde DW. Characterization of a novel HTLV-infected cell
      line. Blood 1984; 64(2) 482-490.

[34] Miyoshi I., Kubonishi I., Sumida M., Hiraki S., Tsubota T., Kimura I., Miyamoto K.,
      Sato J. A novel T-cell line derived from adult T-cell leukemia. Japanese Journal of
      Cancer Research 1980; 71(1) 155-156.

[35] Sugamura K., Fujii M., Kannagi M., Sakitani M., Takeuchi M., Hinuma Y. Cell surface
      phenotypes and expression of viral antigens of various human cell lines carrying hu-
      man T-cell leukemia virus. International Journal of Cancer 1984; 34(2) 221-228.

[36] Yoshida T., Miyagawa E., Yamaguchi K., Kobayashi S., Takahashi Y., Yamashita A.,
      Miura H., Itoyama Y., Yamamoto N. IL-2 independent transformation of a unique
      human T cell line, TY8-3, and its subclones by HTLV-I and -II. International Journal
      of Cancer 2001; 91(1) 99-108.

[37] Nagata K., Ohtani K., Nakamura M., Sugamura K. Activation of endogenous c-fos
      proto-oncogene expression by human T- cell leukemia virus type I-encoded p40 [tax]
      protein in the human T-cell line, Jurkat. Journal of Virology 1989; 63(8) 3220-3226.

[38] Tomita M., Choe J., Tsukazaki T., Mori N. The Kaposi's sarcoma-associated herpesvi-
      rus K-bZIP protein represses transforming growth factor β signaling through interac-
      tion with CREB-binding protein. Oncogene 2004; 23(50) 8272-8281.

[39] Tanaka Y., Yoshida A., Takayama Y., Tsujimoto H., Tsujimoto A., Hayami M., Toza-
      wa H. Heterogeneity of antigen molecules recognized by anti-tax1 monoclonal anti-
      body Lt-4 in cell lines bearing human T cell leukemia virus type I and related
      retroviruses. Japanese Journal of Cancer Research 1990; 81(3) 225-231.

[40] Harrod R., Tang Y., Nicot C., Lu HS., Vassilev A., Nakatani Y., Giam CZ. An exposed
      KID-like domain in human T-cell lymphotropic virus type 1 Tax is responsible for
      the recruitment of coactivators CBP/p300. Molecular and Cellular Biology 1998; 18(9)
      5052-5061.

[41] Matsumoto K., Shibata H., Fujisawa JI., Inoue H., Hakura A., Tsukahara T., Fujii M.
      Human T-cell leukemia virus type 1 Tax protein transforms rat fibroblasts via two
      distinct pathways. Journal of Virology 1997; 71(6) 4445-4451.

[42] Geleziunas R., Ferrell S., Lin X., Mu Y., Cunningham ET, Jr.., Grant M., Connelly
      MA., Hambor JE., Marcu KB., Greene WC. Human T-cell leukemia virus type 1 Tax
      induction of NF-κB involves activation of the IκB kinase a (IKKα) and IKKβ cellular
      kinases. Molecular and Cellular Biology 1998; 18(9) 5157-5165.

[43] Iha H., Kibler KV., Yedavalli VR., Peloponese JM., Haller K., Miyazato A., Kasai T.,
      Jeang KT. Segregation of NF-κB activation through NEMO/IKKγ by Tax and TNFα:

[44] Kajihara M., Sone H., Amemiya M., Katoh Y., Isogai M., Shimano H., Yamada N., Ta-kahashi S. Mouse MafA, homologue of zebrafish somite Maf 1, contributes to the specific transcriptional activity through the insulin promoter. Biochemical and Bio-physical Research Communications 2003; 312(3) 831-842.

[45] Sugita S., Kohno T., Yamamoto K., Imaizumi Y., Nakajima H., Ishimaru T., Matsuya-ma T. Induction of macrophage-inflammatory protein-3α gene expression by TNF dependent NF-κB activation. The Journal of Immunology 2002; 168(11) 5621-5628.

[46] Kataoka K., Fujiwara KT., Noda M., Nishizawa M. MafB, a new Maf family transcrip-tion activator that can associate with Maf and Fos but not with Jun. Molecular and Cellular Biology 1994; 14(11) 7581-7591.

[47] Izuishi K., Kato K., Ogura T., Kinoshita T., Esumi H. Remarkable tolerance of tumor cells to nutrient deprivation: possible new biochemical target for cancer therapy. Cancer Research 2000; 60(21) 6201-6207.

[48] Esumi H., Izuishi K., Kato K., Hashimoto K., Kurashima Y., Kishimoto A., Ogura T., Ozawa T. Hypoxia and nitric oxide treatment confer tolerance to glucose starvation in a 5'-AMP-activated protein kinase-dependent manner. Journal of Biological Chem-istry 2002; 277(36) 32791-32798.

[49] Imamura K., Ogura T., Kishimoto A., Kaminishi M., Esumi H. Cell cycle regulation via p53 phosphorylation by a 5'-AMP activated protein kinase activator, 5-aminoimi-dazole- 4-carboxamide-1-beta-D-ribofuranoside, in a human hepatocellular carcino-ma cell line. Biochemical and Biophysical Research Communications 2001; 287(2) 562-567.

[50] Mori N., Yamada Y., Ikeda S., Yamasaki Y., Tsukasaki K., Tanaka Y., Tomonaga M., Yamamoto N., Fujii M. Bay 11-7082 inhibits transcription factor NF-κB and induces apoptosis of HTLV-I-infected T-cell lines and primary adult T-cell leukemia cells. Blood 2002; 100(5) 1828-1834.

[51] Satou Y., Nosaka K., Koya Y., YasunagaJI.,Toyokuni S., Matsuoka M. Proteasome in-hibitor, bortezomib, potently inhibits the growth of adult T-cell leukemia cells both in vivo and in vitro. Leukemia 2004; 18 1357-1363.

[52] Horie R., Watanabe T., Umezawa K. Blocking NF-κB as a potential strategy to treat adult T-cell leukemia/lymphoma. Drug News & Perspectives 2006; 19(4) 201-209.

[53] Ohsugi T., Kumasaka T., Okada S., Ishida T., Yamaguchi K., Horie R., Watanabe T., Umezawa K. Dehydroxymethylepoxyquinomicin (DHMEQ) therapy reduces tumor formation in mice inoculated with tax-deficient adult T-cell leukemia-derived cell lines. Cancer Letters 2007; 257(2) 206-215.

[54] Peloponese JM, Jr.., Jeang KT. Role for Akt/protein kinase B and activator protein-1 in cellular proliferation induced by the human T-cell leukemia virus type 1 tax oncopro-tein. Journal of Biological Chemistry 2006; 281(13) 8927-8938.

[55] Ikezoe T., Nishioka C., Bandobashi K., Yang Y., Kuwayama Y., Adachi Y., Takeuchi
      T., Koeffler HP., Taguchi H. Longitudinal inhibition of PI3K/Akt/mTOR signaling by
      LY294002 and rapamycin induces growth arrest of adult T-cell leukemia cells. Leuke-
      mia Research 2007; 31(5) 673-682.

[56] JeongSJ.,Dasgupta A., Jung KJ., Um JH., Burke A., Park HU., Brady JN. PI3K/AKT in-
      hibition induces caspase-dependent apoptosis in HTLV-1-transformed cells. Virology
      2008; 370(2) 264-272.

[57] Vivanco I., Sawyers CL. The phosphatidylinositol 3-Kinase AKT pathway in human
      cancer. Nature Reviews Cancer 2002; 2(7) 489-501.

[58] Suzuki A., Kusakai G., Kishimoto A., Shimojo Y., Miyamoto S., Ogura T., Ochiai A.,
      Esumi H. Regulation of caspase-6 and FLIP by the AMPK family member ARK5. On-
      cogene 2004; 23(42) 7067-7075.

[59] Nagata S. Apoptosis by death factor. Cell 1997; 88(3) 355-365.

[60] Ho IC., Hodge MR., Rooney JW.,Glimcher LH. The proto-oncogene c-maf is respon-
      sible for tissue-specific expression of interleukin-4. Cell 1996; 85(7) 973-983.

[61] Inagaki A., Ishida T., Ishii T., Komatsu H., Iida S., Ding J., Yonekura K., Takeuchi S.,
      Takatsuka Y., Utsunomiya A., Ueda R. Clinical significance of serum Th1-, Th2- and
      regulatory T cells-associated cytokines in adult T-cell leukemia/lymphoma: high in-
      terleukin-5 and -10 levels are significant unfavorable prognostic factors. International
      Journal of Cancer 2006; 118(12) 3054-3061.

Permissions

The contributors of this book come from diverse backgrounds, making this book a truly international effort. This book will bring forth new frontiers with its revolutionizing research information and detailed analysis of the nascent developments around the world.

We would like to thank Mariko Tomita, for lending her expertise to make the book truly unique. She has played a crucial role in the development of this book. Without her invaluable contribution this book wouldn't have been possible. She has made vital efforts to compile up to date information on the varied aspects of this subject to make this book a valuable addition to the collection of many professionals and students.

This book was conceptualized with the vision of imparting up-to-date information and advanced data in this field. To ensure the same, a matchless editorial board was set up. Every individual on the board went through rigorous rounds of assessment to prove their worth. After which they invested a large part of their time researching and compiling the most relevant data for our readers. Conferences and sessions were held from time to time between the editorial board and the contributing authors to present the data in the most comprehensible form. The editorial team has worked tirelessly to provide valuable and valid information to help people across the globe.

Every chapter published in this book has been scrutinized by our experts. Their significance has been extensively debated. The topics covered herein carry significant findings which will fuel the growth of the discipline. They may even be implemented as practical applications or may be referred to as a beginning point for another development. Chapters in this book were first published by InTech; hereby published with permission under the Creative Commons Attribution License or equivalent.

The editorial board has been involved in producing this book since its inception. They have spent rigorous hours researching and exploring the diverse topics which have resulted in the successful publishing of this book. They have passed on their knowledge of decades through this book. To expedite this challenging task, the publisher supported the team at every step. A small team of assistant editors was also appointed to further simplify the editing procedure and attain best results for the readers.

Our editorial team has been hand-picked from every corner of the world. Their multi-ethnicity adds dynamic inputs to the discussions which result in innovative outcomes. These outcomes are then further discussed with the researchers and contributors who give their valuable feedback and opinion regarding the same. The feedback is then collaborated with the researches and they are edited in a comprehensive manner to aid the understanding of the subject.

Apart from the editorial board, the designing team has also invested a significant amount of their time in understanding the subject and creating the most relevant covers. They scrutinized every image to scout for the most suitable representation of the subject and create an appropriate cover for the book.

The publishing team has been involved in this book since its early stages. They were actively engaged in every process, be it collecting the data, connecting with the contributors or procuring relevant information. The team has been an ardent support to the editorial, designing and production team. Their endless efforts to recruit the best for this project, has resulted in the accomplishment of this book. They are a veteran in the field of academics and their pool of knowledge is as vast as their experience in printing. Their expertise and guidance has proved useful at every step. Their uncompromising quality standards have made this book an exceptional effort. Their encouragement from time to time has been an inspiration for everyone.

The publisher and the editorial board hope that this book will prove to be a valuable piece of knowledge for researchers, students, practitioners and scholars across the globe.

List of Contributors

Michael Litt
Medical Education Center, Ball State University, Muncie, IN, USA

Bhavita Patel and Ying Li
Department of Bichemistry and Molecular Biology, University of Florida, College of Medicine, Gainesville, FL, USA

Yi Qiu
Shands Cancer Center, University of Florida, College of Medicine, Gainesville, FL, USA
Anatomy and Cell Biology, University of Florida, College of Medicine, Gainesville, FL, USA

Suming Huang
Medical Education Center, Ball State University, Muncie, IN, USA
Shands Cancer Center, University of Florida, College of Medicine, Gainesville, FL, USA

Tsung-Hsien Lin
Department of Pathology, Chi-Mei Medical Center, Tainan, Taiwan

Yen-Chuan Hsieh
Department of Pathology, Chi-Mei Medical Center, Tainan, Taiwan
Department of Biological Science and Technology, Chung Hwa University of Medical Technology, Tainan, Taiwan

Sheng-Tsung Chang
Department of Pathology, Chi-Mei Medical Center, Tainan, Taiwan
Department of Nursing, National Tainan Institute of Nursing, Tainan, Taiwan

Shih-Sung Chuang
Department of Pathology, Chi-Mei Medical Center, Tainan, Taiwan
Department of Pathology, Taipei Medical University, Taipei, Taiwan

Kendle Pryor
Interdepartmental Program in Cell and Molecular Biology, Baylor College of Medicine, Houston, TX, USA

Susan J. Marriott
Interdepartmental Program in Cell and Molecular Biology, Baylor College of Medicine, Houston, TX, USA
Department of Molecular Virology and Microbiology, Baylor College of Medicine, Houston, TX, USA

Hidekatsu Iha
Department of Microbiology, Oita University Faculty of Medicine, Idaigaoka, Hasama, Yufu, Japan

Masao Yamada
GP Biosciences Ltd, -3-3, Azamino-minami, Aoba-ku, Yokohama, Japan

Tahir Latif and John C. Morris
Division of Hematology-Oncology, Department of Medicine, University of Cincinnati, Cincinnati, OH, USA

Makoto Yoshimitsu
Department of Hematology and Immunology, Kagoshima University Hospital, Kagoshima, Japan

Tomohiro Kozako
Department of Biochemistry, Faculty of Pharmaceutical Sciences, Fukuoka University, Fukuoka, Japan

Naomichi Arima
Division of Hematology and Immunology, Center for chronic viral diseases, Graduate School of Medical and Dental Sciences, Kagoshima, Japan
Department of Hematology and Immunology, Kagoshima University Hospital, Kagoshima, Japan

Mariko Tomita
Department of Pathology & Oncology, Graduate School of Medical Science, University of the Ryukyus, Nishihara, Okinawa, Japan

Printed in the USA
CPSIA information can be obtained
at www.ICGtesting.com
JSHW011332221024
72173JS00003B/130